WITHOUT SKIPPING A BEAT:

A Child's Heart Transplant Journey

Kirsten Morgan

WITHOUT SKIPPING A BEAT
A Child's Heart Transplant Journey

Copyright 2019 by Kirsten Morgan
Book Design by R.P. Sprueill
Cover Design by Dick Tumpes

Library of Congress Control Number: 2017943560
ISBN: 978-0-9974990-0-1

BIOGRAPHY & AUTOBIOGRAPHY / Medical / Memoir

Profits from the sale of this book will be donated to
Primary Children's Hospital Foundation.

Published in Golden, Colorado, USA
by Circle Island Press

For Hank the Lionhearted

"In matters of the heart, nothing is true except the improbable."

Madame Germaine de Staël, 1810

Introduction

THIS IS A TALE OF TWO HEARTS. One was healthy, the other tattered beyond repair. Each belonged to a beloved child. Neither would go on beating in its birthplace but would meet at the intersection of their two lives. During this time of terror, and within the constellation of people who surrounded it, lay tenacity, devotion, hope and a large measure of magic. By stirring them all together and letting the flavors blend, a story of many dimensions emerged, one that will carry a different message to each reader.

I recount this unfolding of events from the position of a parent once removed—a grandmother who watched from a short distance as the drama played out on a stage as small as a room and as wide as the world. Just as each child in a family seems to have a different set of parents, each of us involved in this experience observed it through a unique lens. Therefore, my memories reflect my own perspective. However, because the interaction of extended family and friends played a vital role in this tale, I often speak for them as well, for to suggest that I was a primary player is both untrue and unfair to the contributions of many others in this complex support system.

I kept a journal throughout this experience, knowing that the emotional environment would dilute memories with the passage of time. This notebook became the silent voice that heard what couldn't be spoken, the safe place to wander, collapse and revive. Companion, foil, flashlight, it was there in the dark of night and the gray of day as my constant companion, absorbing not only events but also my ever-vacillating relationship with them. It carried details about settings and context, observations of the parents and their evolving process, poetry, favorite quotes—in short, if it came into my mind and stayed awhile, it found its way onto paper. The information contained herein comes primarily from that source but also from extensive interviews with the parents and others intimately involved with the situation, and, of course, from memories so deeply etched that I can pull them up in full descriptive color.

Because my thoughts during this time didn't flow in an organized stream, but gushed, paused, digressed and sprinted in many directions, this narrative is not a smooth path. It is instead a collection of anecdotes, impressions and reflections experienced from a slight distance but with a visceral emotional engagement.

May this story become a guide for those who, regardless of circumstance or detail, make their way through great challenge without a map. It's a lonely and terrifying journey but one that can open vistas, provide epiphanies and bring to the surface a deep and unequivocal love for the gifts in strange wrappings that appear on our doorsteps during these times of fear and wonder.

Kirsten Morgan

ONE

"Wrapp'd and confounded in a thousand fears..."

William Shakespeare

I FIRST MET HANK IN A HOSPITAL ROOM, two weeks old and abruptly transformed from a healthy baby into a medical conundrum. Tubed, tangled and tethered, he held onto life by a thread, with eyes closed and the beeps and whistles of mechanized monitors as his lullaby. Leaning very close, his father whispered into the boy's ear. As those words filled the space between them, Hank awoke, turned his head and looked into his dad's eyes as if to affirm the truth he had just heard. I never asked, but my son might have said, "You will live and you will grow and you will be whole again. I'm your father and you have my promise."

Henry Bridgeman, to be called "Hank," was brand-new but already tarnished by a harsh reality. The boy who would rock our world had begun his strange and magnificent journey.

His crib sat like a small shrine in the center of the great, white room, surrounded by technological and pharmaceutical miracles of western medicine. Potions seeped in through his spidery blood vessels, and machines tracked measurements and functions while Hank lay unmoving in the midst of organized chaos. We humans, helpless and hopeful, created the second circle, whispering, watching, wondering at the machinations that kept him alive, an orb of audience that existed in some suspended time and space. We floated without markers through the minutes and hours, remembering to take an occasional deep breath.

Hank had cleaved from his mother on the appointed day and hour, entering with grace but carrying a secret. Wearing the cloak of health, he didn't reveal the incongruity that lay buried within his chest. Alert and engaged with his new family, he rarely cried and he nursed with vigor—the baby everyone hopes for. Ned and Annie, his proud parents, were relieved to know their family had been completed. Two-year-old Georgia was already planning to groom her new brother into a personal pet.

And then, two weeks later, this healthy child began to turn a bit blue around the lips and extremities. He didn't want to nurse, was cold to the touch and became tachypnic—the first of many new words that would quickly enter our vocabularies—as he started rapid, shallow breathing. His terrified parents rushed him to the emergency room of Primary Children's Hospital near their home in Salt Lake City, where they learned that his temperature had fallen to ninety-five degrees. A team of doctors and a deluge of tests presented a host of possibilities—meningitis, a viral attack, cardiomyopathy, encephalitis. They just didn't know. By now Hank was in full-blown cardiac failure.

Annie overheard medical personnel in the emergency room: "We've got a baby—it looks bad, really bad." Hank was soon transferred to the Pediatric Intensive Care Unit (PICU), but his frantic parents, with frightened and confused Georgia in tow, paced a private waiting room as a medical team tried to stabilize their son. Ned, an anesthesiology resident at the University of Utah Medical School, understood the gravity of the situation from a physician's standpoint;

Annie knew only that her beautiful baby was suffering and she couldn't be there to hold him close. Upon finally being paged, after several hours with little information, they ran to the PICU and found Hank splayed in his hospital crib—intubated and unconscious, with lines running into his body from top of head to foot, and surrounded by a buzz of support staff. The parents could only stroke his cheek and repeat to each other the big lie that everything was going to be all right.

The next morning, a team of specialists held a meeting with Ned and Annie. More refined examination had finally revealed a condition whose name was as long as his tiny foot—Left Ventricular Noncompaction. The ventricle wasn't pumping efficiently, possibly a congenital anomaly or perhaps the result of a coxsackie B virus. Since he knew it could cause this condition, Ned had requested lab tests to see if the virus might be a factor, and the results confirmed its presence. However, it was impossible to know whether this was the origin of Hank's cardiomyopathy or simply a strange coincidence. At this point, the cause was far less important than immediate treatment. A cure was impossible. The heart would not heal itself.

His only chance for survival was a transplant. But, doctors explained that the chances of finding a healthy heart to fit such a small recipient were miniscule and the surgery extraordinarily risky. They pointed out, with the gravity of their training as scientists, that, even if those circumstances were surmounted, his lifestyle and that of the family would always be compromised by his severe limitations. With greatest compassion, the doctors offered the option of taking Hank home and simply holding him close for the remaining few days of his life, discontinuing medications and letting nature take its course.

Still in shock but thinking clearly, the new parents didn't pause long before instructing the medical magicians to do everything in their power to keep this little guy afloat. They would take their chances on consequences and no interruption of glorious future plans mattered. This young couple, who spent every free moment engaged in outdoor sports, travel or adventure, tossed away possibilities of that life for their family without a backward glance.

Annie's parents, Bruce and Paula, dropped everything when they heard the news and raced from their home in Ketchum, Idaho, to Salt Lake City, a five-hour drive. Along with my daughter, Bryn, I left Denver early the next morning and arrived at the family's home to find them and Annie's brother, George, a graduate student at the University of Utah, all looking stunned and speaking in quiet tones. In the living room was an empty baby carrier. Upon seeing it, I burst into tears. Georgia crawled onto my lap, stroked my face and assured me, "It's going to be all right, Nanny. Hank will be home soon," and then burrowed as I wrapped her in my arms.

Hank was failing fast. I had packed my bags for only a few days, but would stay as long as necessary. However, Bruce, Paula and I weren't the only ones to rush to Salt Lake. In a show of uncommon loyalty, Ned's friend, Jason, upon hearing the news, immediately flew from Portland without announcement and came directly to the hospital in the middle of the night. The parents, too exhausted to stay, had gone home for a few hours' rest and their friend couldn't be admitted to the intensive care area without a family member present. Not wanting to disturb Ned and Annie, he spent the cold night trying to sleep in his rental car in the hospital parking garage, hoping he hadn't arrived too late to see Hank and provide scaffolding for Ned. His visit, spontaneous and difficult, was gratefully received as an act of deep friendship, the first of countless others in the months to come.

The word "transplant" whispered through the gathering of extended family, but we simply rejected it as impossible. Perhaps the diagnosis was inaccurate. Perhaps he would miraculously recover. The idea of a transplant—so huge, so terrifying—just couldn't find a place in our heads. Yet the doctors gently but repeatedly broached it, until that possibility finally lodged on the far edges of our psyches. It became the word that couldn't be spoken, the threat that stuck in our throats.

Within a few days, however, Ned and Annie fully understood that it was their only option and signed papers for the procedure, to go into effect when necessary. If everything worked optimally, and Hank responded to the host of medications, the doctors hoped to keep him alive long enough to gain some weight and strength, increasing his chances for a successful surgery. He wouldn't be listed until his body was as ready as a tiny, weak vessel could be.

Meanwhile, Georgia, wise as a crone, refused the crisis and assigned herself the role of jester for the gathered family members. As tears leaked, she danced. As low voices shared fears, she stood on her head. And, when our words failed, she sang to us. Her presence spoke of hope and possibility. She demanded little and seemed grateful just to be participating in the mystery and excitement of this turn of events.

I began a self-designed crash course in Heart 101, suddenly needing to know everything about the physiology, development, function and anything else that might increase my understanding of this engine that drives all other systems. Among other things, I learned that the heart initiates its tiny spark of pulse when the fetus is just three weeks old, the first organ to form and announce its existence. In a process known as "spontaneous depolarization," channels deep inside the cells start to leak sodium. This in turn initiates a trade of calcium and potassium, and that exchange creates the beginnings of an electrical current that becomes a beat. In a fetus much smaller than the period at the end of this sentence, cells that will shape the heart speak in the body's first voice, sending a pulse pattern that will last a lifetime. In utero photos reveal the heart as a huge, red lump on the chest, appearing to be almost outside the body but covered by a thin veil of skin. This fist of flesh seems to open and close as it sends messages even the brain hasn't begun to understand.

Both Ned's and Annie's extended families had always been healthy—few serious illnesses, good habits, positive outcomes. Most elders had lived to a ripe old age. We almost believed ourselves immune to the slings and arrows that bedeviled other families, although, deep down, we knew life didn't work that way. So, when this tiny product of strong parents and a textbook pregnancy presented with a serious heart anomaly, we were stunned. It's surprising to look back at our credulity, but we simply had limited experience in such things. In support of Ned and Annie, we rallied in record time but were still terrified by the prospect of a transplant with all its complex conceptual baggage. Most difficult to process was the knowledge that someone else had to leave this planet in order for our child to stay. We couldn't create a context to take in something of this magnitude as even a remote possibility, so we chose to believe a miracle was about to happen and Hank would slowly recover. But, while all other heads dove for the sand, Ned and Annie marched forward with eyes wide open.

Cardiologists explained that the walls of Hank's left ventricle resembled cheesecloth, shot with holes that kept it from pumping efficiently; this critical chamber simply couldn't do its job. Yet, in ways mysterious and stunning, the stew of medications that now swam through his bloodstream could keep that small pump pulsing. Ten tubes and lines went in, or were taped to, his tiny body. His head, arms, chest, hands and feet were plugged into life support as monitors beeped and scrawled their enigmatic language.

Most of us take the heart for granted—the perpetual motion machine that pulls all systems together, the origin of life force, a maze of vessels and functions designed with elegance of purpose that fuels a system of continuous delivery and return. Any science teacher can describe the heart as an exquisite engine composed of upper chambers (atria) and lower chambers (ventricles), an organ that labors without rest from the first flicker of embryonic life until its owner takes a final breath. With this continuous tympanic rhythm, the body's symphony can render beautiful music; without it, all other systems play out of tune. The physiology is simple: the atria contract at the same time, pushing blood down into the ventricles—right atrium to right ventricle, left atrium to left ventricle. The right ventricle sends its flow to the lungs for oxygenation; the left ventricle sends it to the far reaches of the body. The heart relaxes for a brief moment. Blood then fills the heart again and the entire process repeats.

I came to a new appreciation of the word "ventricle," usually used to describe a cavity in the heart or brain. Although it's a hollow space, it's not empty, but serves as a space-saver, either for blood or cerebral fluid—that allows for expansion and contraction. This word, both in reality and concept, began to creep into my thinking and soon became metaphor: place between, a storage space, eminent domain to be used as needed for the greater good. Or, in another application, it became a new place in my own mind, where I could swell and shrivel while accepting the enormity of this process. I moved into a philosophical ventricle, where truth could no longer be contained and everything could shape-shift in the blink of an eye. And I eventually found a bit of comfort there.

Surprisingly, Hank stabilized, roused and then did his version of a rally. Within just three days, the "t" word lost some of its power as Hank gained his. He was no longer a baby on the verge of departure, but instead a symbol of possibility as he responded to medications and slowly came back to life. His eyes were open much of the time and he followed movement with seeming interest. We didn't let down our guard, but most of us allowed a few deeper breaths, and, perhaps, a bit more sleep as we tried to calm our worst fears into some manageable package. We even went out to dinner and managed a bit of conversation unrelated to the topic that dominated our thoughts.

Although he was initially expected to stay in the hospital for at least six months, if he lived that long, Hank was discharged just eleven days after arriving in the ER, accompanied by a satchel of drugs—thirteen in all—to be administered at home with great care at precise times. Who knew digitalis and Viagra had applications in treating a child's raggedy heart? But they, along with other wonder drugs, stepped in and took charge like drill sergeants with a new recruit. Any deviation from schedule was potentially deadly. These potions, with a language of their own, would speak to his tiny body, delivering precise instructions to each system. Because of his medical training, Ned could assess any changes, and the family lived only ten minutes from the Primary Children's Hospital emergency room. Annie's devotion was without question, and their son would be safe from the germs that lurk in hospital halls. No one, including doctors, saw a future beyond each passing day, but these quotidian markers were small gifts and the family held tightly to each one. Hank had made an amazing recovery relative to initial expectations, but we now accepted the fact that he was still a little boy with a malfunctioning heart. We also knew it couldn't, under any circumstances, perform its intended function, nor could it heal itself.

I remember watching myself during this time, still living in a place of wild hope when there was no evidence to support that naïve position. I couldn't find another path at that point, nor could I allow myself to wander into frightening territory. Denial, said to be the first stage of grief. Over time, I came to understand that both hope and apprehension can be held simultaneously, with neither negating the other. In those early days, however, I went on wild roller coaster rides of emotion, coming to an occasional stop and then careening off again through a world let loose. How could I prepare for the great unknown? Should I temper my love with defenses against an outcome too chilling to name? Where could I find relief, or was it even to be found?

All extended family members and close friends opened to a spectrum of possibilities from bad to worse, but, like a troupe of actors, we painted courage on our public faces in a mad scramble of mutual protection, falling into our dark holes only in private moments. These tricks of mind kept us sane, providing balance and allowing the disguise of normalcy to cover terror. And even that emotion gradually lost its power as we surrendered attempts at control.

When Hank returned home from the hospital, it was as though a miniature potentate had taken up residence. Everything shifted around his protection and maintenance. Each act became deliberate, each response considered. Nothing could be left to chance, and so his life was minutely regulated. At the same time, his parents knew their family had to live as though this new guest was a commoner, so they struggled to maintain balance while guarding against every potential danger. Georgia played the perfect supporting role, yielding most of her needs to his and somehow understanding that she no longer held the spotlight. She watched her brother throughout the day, still trying to figure out where he had been all that time and why he looked like any other baby but still needed special attention. "Daddy, Hank keeps wiggling his arms and legs. Maybe there's a bug under his shirt!"

Annie had placed her teaching career on hold so she could devote her time and energy to parenting, especially since Ned, who usually put in eighty-hour weeks at the hospital, was rarely home. She had leaped into full-time mothering as to the manner born and loved turning in the direction of domesticity, assuming she would return one day to her other career. Because of this decision, she was available to multitask in hyperdrive, not only mothering an active two-year-old and a very sick baby, but also running a household. When he was home, Ned jumped into action instead of trying to catch a few extra hours of sleep. With relentless patience, they did what needed to be done, their own needs now low on the priority list.

Medications were to be taken in precise measure at exact times to keep Hank's body stable. Interactions with people who might challenge his compromised immune system with their own illnesses were to be avoided at all costs. His caregivers, relatives and friends were constantly attuned to his condition. And all of this needed to happen in the context of a normal family life in order to protect their sanity and keep both kids in a place of emotional safety.

Things fell into place, and the exceptional became the accustomed. As days gathered into weeks, Annie's triangulation was home, doctor and grocery store. Frequent trips to the clinic measured Hank's vital signs. Monthly EKGs and chest x-rays monitored chest cavity changes and potential fluid accumulation. This was as much a part of her life as any other regular activity, but each visit was accompanied by a shiver of trepidation as she wondered what change those numbers and images might reveal. Medications were added and subtracted, dosages finely tuned in response to the latest measurements. Ned, when work kept him from being at the appointment, waited by the phone for the latest news.

A continual state of sleep-deprived alertness defined the parents' hours as they listened for Hank's every sound during the day and checked on him regularly throughout the night. But dividing time between him and his sister, while trying to stay upright, both physically and emotionally, didn't appear to take a toll. If anything, the parents seemed to grow stronger as each new fear sought, and was refused, entry into their psyches.

Ned carried the burden of performance expectations along with constant trepidation as he tried to imagine the future. Sleepless nights at work became sleepless nights at home. He had the strength of someone who faces life and death situations daily and somehow finds equilibrium, but fear was still his constant companion. He knew his wife was strong, but how could she possibly hold up under continuous pressure while also processing her version of deep anxiety? How could he come home at night and look into his son's eyes while knowing what he knew about his boy's probable future? How could he allow a bond that might soon be severed?

The human spirit is a powerful vessel with bottomless resources. Through pure will, Ned and Annie held on tightly to each other. They developed a synergy in which each fed and sustained the other, even with little hope for respite. And so they moved from past and future into the present—this moment, this hour. In this place, they found a version of comfort and became skilled at balancing relative stability with an unknown outcome.

They weren't completely confined and removed from social interaction. Both parents continued a modified exercise routine by switching out childcare—short hikes, taking a run around the neighborhood or dropping by the rec center. But, instead of climbing rock cliffs in the canyons above their home or going mountain biking for hours, Ned now built a climbing wall in his garage and rode his exercise bike in the basement. Annie ran around the neighborhood with the kids in a double stroller. Friends dropped by or visited in the yard, but all knew to keep a wide distance if they or their kids showed the slightest sign of illness. Frequent phone calls from family members and friends around the country kept the parents grounded and in touch with their network of supporters. National Public Radio played throughout each day, bringing the world into their living room.

They prepared special meals, created excuses for small celebrations at home, played games, read books and, in most ways, functioned like any other family. Annie, already an immaculate housekeeper, scrubbed every touchable surface with a disinfectant and kept the entire house swept, mopped and sterilized, a never-ending task. Industrial-sized bottles of hand sanitizers were always available for use by anyone entering the house. It worked, and, with modifications, family life wasn't so different from those of other families.

As Hank's grandmother, I occupied the position all grandparents come to accept, that of strong supporter but peripheral player. In this role, we who have spent decades as linchpins now move aside, regardless of the situation, and become parents once removed, a response not difficult, just different. I desperately wanted to know everything, but waited to be brought into the information loop if and when the parents deemed it necessary. Over the next months, I spent as much time as possible with the family, but, with 500 miles between our homes, these trips carried personal challenges, both for me and for my husband, Dave, who was dealing with his own medical issues. However, I couldn't stay away; they needed me and I needed to be there. Recently retired, I had the luxury of discretionary time, so I frequently grabbed books on CDs from the library, jumped into my faithful car and headed west. By helping with laundry, driving, cooking and other daily chores, I hoped to buy Annie some relief.

All right, I admit it. I now surprised myself by seeking auguries, having retreated into my reptilian brain with attendant diminishment of logic. A vivid dream? Tea leaves? A heart-shaped cloud or the face of Jesus on a piece of toast? At this point, I might have embraced anything as a divination. I've always prided myself on staying planted in reality, but this kind of perpetual balancing act eventually does strange things to emotional equilibrium. Surely a small sign from some invisible but all-knowing source wouldn't be too much to ask? I remained alert, but few messages appeared.

Heart. Heartful, heartache, heartbreak, hearten, hearty. An open heart, closed heart, hard heart, warm heart. *Coeur*, core, courage. A crucial component of our expressive language. I was suddenly surrounded by metaphors, with each carrying a beat, a rhythm, a message. The word frequently found its way into my vocabulary; I drew hearts in margins; I touched my chest when thinking about Hank or discussing his status with others. In times of greatest challenge, cliché became reality and aphorisms sprang to life, losing triteness to become profound.

I know Ned and Annie often slipped into Hank's room during his sleeping hours, both day and night, to watch his chest rise and fall and have silent conversations with their son. I also tiptoed into his dreaming space during visits. My hand on my grandson's chest, I tried to connect with a higher energy that might join with ours to bring him the strength to survive. I believe he knew each of us was there and that his body rallied under our touch and intention. Whether or not it was true, this consistent connection, almost a meditation, was critically important to all of us.

Fall slowly faded, and fear yielded to watchfulness. The family found its rhythm and slipped more easily into a cadence of four heartbeats pulsing as one. Annie, ever the conscious keeper of her children's emotional health, continued to yield her personal life to their needs, spending every spare moment with Georgia while holding Hank as close as possible throughout each day. She drank him in, memorized every detail of his body, felt his warmth, smelled his fragrance, stroked, cooed and sang. Ned continued to spend every spare and rare minute with his family—sharing chores, playing with the kids and rarely letting them out of his sight or touch. He, too, held Hank like a puppy, feeling his warmth, storing every detail of his essence. The act of capturing in memory someone who may soon depart is an exercise both in mindfulness and unease, but it was their great solace. Hank melted into his Mom and Dad as though their contours had been designed for just this circumstance. He filled their space and they filled his. Love doesn't get more pure and simple.

Georgia, busy as a hummingbird, engaged herself in endless projects, loved having books read repeatedly, helped her mom cook, asked a thousand questions and displayed other typical two-year-old behaviors. The creativity that would later capture so much of her energy had already begun to show up in dozens of amazing and frustrating ways. She gathered boxes, feathers, leaves, strings and paper to concoct imaginary scenarios, always peopled with characters invented on the spot. Nothing was to be moved or disassembled, although she consistently flew on to other projects while wanting their predecessors to stay on the dining room table, or splayed across a couch cushion. She talked to Hank incessantly, oblivious to the fact that he didn't answer. However, even at that early age, he fixed his eyes on her while she chattered, so she was undeterred by his lack of response. She lived in the world of her own creation, but was very much a participant in the family web.

Thanksgiving arrived and friends from Denver, Spider and Annie, along with their sons, came to Salt Lake City. They swooped into the house, loaded with all the trappings for a feast, and set to work. Soon, Georgia and Hank were royally entertained, as the bigger boys brought Georgia into their games while Hank watched. Spider took Ned skiing, climbing and hiking. Meanwhile, his Annie took charge of the kitchen while our Annie relaxed and took a few deep breaths.

Several years earlier, while they were in college, Spider and Ned, along with close friends, Jason and Bryan, had worked together at a mountain sports store in Boulder, Colorado. Their jobs gave them discounts on climbing equipment and took them on escapades that kept them on the edge of danger and their mothers at a perpetual level of high anxiety. Ice and rock climbing, backcountry skiing, kayaking, bicycling, and anything else that required sweat and challenge, occupied all their free hours and also bonded their friendship forever. They called themselves "The Band."

Though now separated by geography, this boundary-testing gang of four had stuck together in the ensuing years, so reaching out to each other in a time of need was an extension of what they'd always done. In the group, they always referred to Ned as "The Guardian," the one who, when they entered dangerous climbing or skiing territory, kept them safe by reminding them of boundaries and common sense. Now they stayed by his side, in person or by telephone, to guard the guardian as he traveled through territory more perilous than any of them had ever encountered in the wilderness.

As winter slowly passed, numbers, those cold markers of Hank's progress, vacillated enough to keep his parents on edge but stayed within the realm of relative safety. Doctors became as familiar as family; needle pricks were part of life, as were frequent trips to small bright rooms filled with gentle strangers who poked and prodded him. The doctors were perplexed. Nothing about his condition seemed consistent with their training or experience. He wasn't supposed to make progress, but he was doing so. He shouldn't have met developmental milestones, but he did. His numbers, the algorithmic legerdemain that measured left ventricle blood volume, defied all expectations as they stayed low but steady instead of gradually sinking into oblivion. However, Hank was often tired and his appetite couldn't be cajoled beyond survival level; at three months, he had grown in length but weighed only nine pounds.

Hank maintained a low but steady level of stamina. Determined to be in the world as fully as possible, he summoned all his energy in order to participate. In time, and on time, he learned to crawl and his borders slowly crumbled. Now the master of his movements, Hank crept through the house, exploring each cranny with diligence and intensity. He picked up or touched everything within reach, a puff of lint getting as much attention as a toy. But, instead of fleeting concentration, he spent long minutes in close examination, a scientist always on the verge of discovery in this new world at his fingertips.

This child, whose heart pumped at about twenty-five percent of capacity, also loved jumping up and down in the bouncing seat that hung in a doorway, laughing and babbling as Annie went about her tasks and Georgia created a flurry of excitement. But best of all were stroller adventures. He came to full attention at the prospect of exploring that outside world where garbage trucks gulped and gigantic yellow machines dug holes. Everything fascinated Hank.

The kids and I loved to tell and hear stories. I regularly concocted tales based on events of the day, while Georgia added details along the way and Hank listened wide-eyed as these wild adventures flew out of my imagination. I also told them my versions of old classic favorites, like Goldilocks and the Three Bears, Cinderella, and Georgia's all-time favorite, the Three Little Pigs. One day I was carrying eight-month-old Hank while recounting the story of pigs who left home to find their fortune, encountering the big, bad wolf along the way. Of course I couldn't just tell the tale, but had to get into character as well, using high squealing voices for the pigs and a rough, raspy, low and loud voice for the wolf. When I came to "I'LL HUFF AND I'LL PUFF AND I'LL BLOW THE HOUSE DOWN," I heard whimpering sounds from Hank and worried that I'd frightened him. However, looking down, I saw that he was laughing so hysterically that he could hardly catch his breath. All of us whooped in delighted relief that Hank's sense of humor was tuned to absurdity.

Although he nursed, as much for nourishment as for connection, Hank's appetite continued to be restricted by fatigue and

19

side effects from medication. His parents did everything they could to get him to eat some baby food, or nibble on crackers, but nothing tasted good to him and he ingested only a few extra calories each day. By spring, his beanpole body couldn't do its best work without additional nourishment, so a feeding tube was inserted, taped to his cheek and gently threaded into his nostril and down into his stomach. Each night, while Hank slept, a bag hung from an IV pole next to his bed and dripped supplemental formula into his tummy. He didn't gain much weight, but as he grew in length, he managed to pick up a few extra pounds.

Hank had an interesting habit. He closely observed every event unfolding in front of him. He studied people, listened to conversations, and seemed fascinated with all forms of human interaction. It was as though his self-assigned job was to collect as much information from as many people and situations as possible. He didn't demand attention, as if this would diminish his determination to gather the world into a manageable package. In an adult, it would be called mindfulness; in a child, it was unusual, but nothing about Hank's way in the world surprised us at this point. He lived in his own little universe, removed in every way from expectation while puttering through each day in his unique rhythm.

We decided his hair stood on end because so much brain activity was happening just beneath it. Regardless of the reason, two inches of hair, unresponsive to attempts at taming it, gave him the look of perpetual curiosity. Even more fascinating were eyes that could only be described as extraordinary—unusually large, blue, framed with long lashes. He seemed to look right into the essence of each person who gained his attention, and on many occasions a brief encounter—with a checkout clerk or someone who paused to coo at him—resulted in a complete stranger declaring, "Wow, this kid has amazing eyes!"

In more respects than anyone would have expected, he was a normal kid—fussy at times, protective of his interests, a tester of boundaries and, considering his physical condition, a full participant in nearly all aspects of family life. No one tiptoed around him or treated him differently. He yelled, cried and laughed at appropriate times and became adept at handling an older sister who wasn't above teasing and manipulation.

While Annie and Ned became relatively comfortable with their son's tenuous way in the world, I, hundreds of miles away much of the time, found myself periodically sinking into despair as my imagination scampered through an ever-shifting film of scenarios. How does one walk at the edge of a precipice for months on end without yielding to a measure of madness? I'm convinced, without any research to support my instincts, that one of the brain's finest self-protective mechanisms is the ability to place ongoing fear in its own compartment while the body continues to put one foot in front of the other. To sustain an extreme level of negative anticipation is to lose life along the way, so it becomes a companion whose company isn't welcomed but whose daily appearance becomes habituated and thus manageable. It's a form of grief, but, because the outcome is unknown, it has a different face and a separate set of rules. Seneca wrote, "We suffer more from imagination than reality." It became my quest, and in time my liberation, to steer my thinking away from dread and replace it with other possibilities.

No one else, on either side of the family, had seen Hank in person, but all felt such a strong bond that this invisible boy was a constant, imagined presence in their lives. He remained a shadow, an image in photos, the subject of endless stories—all weak substitutes for seeing, hearing and touching a real, live boy. Without any of us intending this outcome, he almost achieved mythic status, and experiencing this child through a personal encounter became a fixation for many of our altruistic clan. But it was not to be, not yet, perhaps never. I considered the possibility that he would come into and leave this world without ever joining the great groups of relatives on both sides who loved and supported each other through good times and bad.

Although we were raised Catholic, my siblings and I pretty much eschewed organized religion. Our generation had its fill while growing up and, although we exposed our kids to a quasi-Catholic tradition, we found ourselves loath to expect of our children what we couldn't generate ourselves. But we're not without a strong spiritual sensibility, and were each able to access this in our own way as crisis turned into a way of life. Our version of prayer, different for each of us, became a lifestyle, not as part of a bedtime routine, but more as a continual consciousness. The family on both sides—grandparents, cousins, aunts, uncles—took up this cause with generosity of spirit and attention. My sister Kate thought she had become an atheist until she found herself on her knees beseeching the God she had abandoned. Family members not only kept in close touch with us, but also sent the message out to their circles of friends and acquaintances. Pastors announced Hank's story from the pulpit. Many other groups took him under their spiritual wing. Soon it seemed as though hundreds, perhaps thousands of people were part of a broad network of supporters. "I'm praying for you," became a common assurance, one that left cliché to become a tenuous thread of hope.

None of us was drawn back into a church, but none remained unmoved by the energy that came our way via prayer. Others in the family agreed with me that at times a force seemed to envelop every space, an experience so palpable we had to question whether our overactive imaginations had created it or whether we were truly sensing the power of subtle energy in whatever form it was being sent. We felt lightened, suspended, even buzzing, as though we were captured in a great balloon of good will and endless, crazy hope. We'll never know whether it kept Hank alive or nurtured our spirits enough to keep our balance during tremulous times. Actually, we believe it did both, and we will be forever grateful for, and astonished by, the hundreds of unknown strangers who cared enough to send healing energy our way.

Hank's family lived in the middle of a very strong Latter Day Saints community, with a Ward Church just down the block. As though transported back to Centerville in the 1950's, we all watched the sidewalks periodically fill with churchgoers, dressed up and often holding hands, strolling to and from their place of worship. Ned and Annie had forged strong friendships with some of their Mormon neighbors and had been accepted by others as friendly outliers. Although we weren't part of the official community, as I pushed Hank up and down the streets in a stroller, people from blocks around stopped to inquire about his progress and reassure me that they continued to keep him in their prayers. These were total strangers, people who had never, as far as I knew, seen him or me. And yet they somehow knew who he was and cared enough to reach out, with all borders erased and the protection of a small and fragile life the only thing that mattered.

We took lots of photographs of Hank—hundreds, maybe thousands—but none of us talked about why. Every expression required capture and each carried a slice of life. Perhaps, pasted together one dark day, they would bring him into our presence if he couldn't be there in person. Most people become adept at culling digital photos that don't quite measure up, but we kept every single one, as though discarding anything might suggest a future casting away. Single, recorded seconds stitching together a life provided a different sense of comfort, and we collected them with passion.

As spring returned and temperatures rose, the constant danger of lurking germs diminished. Georgia had friends over to play; neighbors dropped by more frequently; Annie took the kids farther afield—to the zoo, museums and restaurants—always protective of Hank. His world expanded again when he learned to walk and now, in summer's warmth, it included the entire back yard, where bugs, rocks and flowers required intense study. Several of Ned's and Annie's friends came with their kids to celebrate his first birthday in July. They must have joined us in wondering what lay ahead for this little guy with the mysterious heart whose function still seemed to hold steady, although weak and very tenuous. No one could predict or imagine his possible future. so we still allowed ourselves to wander unwittingly into the world of ludicrous hope, based on nothing but a quasi-belief in some kind of cosmic intercession. He seemed to be filling out and putting on weight; he looked healthier than he had in months. We almost convinced ourselves his heart might change its mind. But we weren't that naive, and at a deep level we knew the worst was surely yet to come.

On a beautiful late summer day in the Rocky Mountains, my son, Bridge, and I climbed to the top of the world, to the Continental Divide Trail high above Colorado's Berthoud Pass. At 12,500 feet elevation, this treeless environment, with strewn rocks and soil-hugging flowers, brought a kind of peace that we very much needed. As we looked around at mountain peaks in every direction and the pure elegance of the setting, Bridge suggested we build a shrine, a tangible tribute to Hank in which we could not only put our physical efforts but also insert our hopes that a greater universe was part of his journey. Setting ourselves to the task before afternoon storms rolled in, we gathered rocks, most of them volcanic in that particular spot, and shaped them into a rough pyramid, topping it with a triangular stone. We named it a holy place, one that, as we added rocks on future climbs, would continue to grow and speak its own language.

Each time thereafter when I hiked to that aerie, I looked for a rock along the way that carried the approximate shape of a heart. Interestingly, one always appeared and I placed it among the rest, then paused to remember the sense of peace this small monument had first provided. Its sturdiness against the wailing storms of winter provided yet another symbolic reminder of the strength we continued to seek, a tangible metaphor in an unstable world.

A September family reunion in the mountains above Salt Lake City brought a sense of relaxation we hadn't allowed ourselves in the fourteen months since the ordeal began. In his dad's safe arms, Hank ventured into the hotel swimming pool. He loved hikes, tucked into a backpack that provided a broader view of the world. And of course he watched and listened to countless conversations from his position at the side of the action. He looked good—a bit plumper, with bright eyes and pink cheeks.

But our delight was not to last. The elevation, in combination with other unknown factors, sent his attenuated heart into a tailspin. Shortly after his return home, all of those shaky numeric markers crashed like the stock market and along with them, our unfounded hope. He retained fluids and his carotid artery pulsed like a bass drum. He gasped and then held his breath in a futile attempt to bring oxygen into his system. The weight gain that had given us so much hope had been due to fluid retention; his weakening heart just couldn't pump enough blood to his kidneys. Soon he was back in the hospital, and the entire testing scenario returned. The medical team adjusted medications, looked at numbers, and tried to figure out what to do next to keep him going.

But they knew one thing for sure, and this time the doctors didn't beat around the bush—a transplant was his only chance for survival. It had to happen, and soon. We immediately shifted mental gears toward an outcome that we now fervently desired. It became the magic bullet, the miracle that would buy time. A few months, perhaps even a few years. Longer? Wishes fluttered around possibility, but too much wishful thinking almost brought guilt into the equation. What reason did we have to trust that Hank would be one of the few lucky ones? Why did we believe he might actually get a heart, survive and, possibly, even thrive? However, hope always flickers after the flames of logic die, and it was our only remaining resource.

Hank eventually stabilized enough to allow us to relax a bit. Because his doctor believed he would fare as well at home as at the hospital, he was dismissed from the ER as soon as his meds were carefully calibrated. Georgia was now in preschool so Annie had a bit of extra time to support this little boy as he struggled mightily to navigate his small world. He had to stop and lie down awhile on the floor as he made the long trip from living room to kitchen, a distance of fifteen feet. A feeding tube once again provided nourishment for a child still too exhausted to do more than pick at his food. Because he was now actively listed as a transplant candidate, a new scenario was added to the others—waiting and wondering whether a heart might actually find its way to this desperate family.

TWO

"Now is the winter of our discontent..."

William Shakespeare

HANK'S NAME WENT ON THE NATIONAL TRANSPLANT LIST, but was so far down that his chances of surviving until his number came up were slim. Then, in early November, during a trip to the zoo in a stroller, this frail little boy couldn't even hold up his head. Annie once again rushed him to the Children's Hospital emergency room, where Ned soon joined them. Because Hank was now sinking fast, the doctors knew there was no time to waste and admitted him to the Pediatric Intensive Care Unit, where, by administering a powerful medication with massive side effects, they would try to keep his heart beating until a replacement became available. Not only was he too sick to stay home, but as a hospital patient, he was also moved automatically to top priority status as a transplant candidate.

Dave and I had let down our guard enough to take a three-week trip to Eastern Europe during which we had only limited news from home, so we weren't aware of the severity of Hank's changed condition. We arrived back in Denver exhausted, and I looked forward to a week or so of recovery, after which there would be a return trip to Utah. That evening Ned called to report that Hank was hospitalized and things looked grim. I snatched a few hours of sleep, then threw some clothes into the car and, fueled by caffeine, sped to Salt Lake City, prepared to stay as long as necessary.

I moved in with the family, Annie and Ned moved into Hank's hospital room and Georgia moved once again into her strength, pulling up a level of grace virtually unheard of in a three-year-old, as her mother and father virtually disappeared and I provided an interesting but inadequate substitute. These days were difficult at first, and I was often exhausted, but my challenges paled next to those of Hank's parents. Eventually, I, too, fell into a comfortable rhythm, feeling useful at last after several months of helplessness.

The day after Hank was admitted, Ned developed severe nerve pain in his cheek. His right eye throbbed and he couldn't close it. His face seemed to droop a bit and his smile was frozen on one side. The diagnosis was easy but frightening—he had Bell's Palsy, a condition in which the cranial nerve becomes constricted as it passes through a narrow channel behind the ear. Bell's has many possible causes, but, in this case, stress was the assumed culprit, a physical manifestation of an emotional maelstrom. It usually heals in a few weeks when the contributing situation resolves, but in this case, as Hank's future swayed in tenuous balance, there would be no relief from dark, cold fear.

Ned learned to live with his lingering condition, going about life as usual. For the first several weeks, he couldn't blink or close his eye, so he used drops to keep it moist and found a substance to glue it closed at night. The facial paralysis gradually improved, but vestiges remained. Ned never mentioned it and never complained, accepting it as a manifestation of a situation so paralyzing that his body shrieked in the only language available.

Annie discarded any pretense of the life she had known and dove into her new existence with characteristic determination. Since I was there, she quickly made a big decision. By taking up residence in

Hank's room, she knew he would rarely be alone in this scary place and was equally certain that, should something go suddenly awry, she would be there to respond immediately. Ned also moved into the room whenever possible, giving precious hours to his son and allowing Annie to slip away. Everything else assumed a distant second place in their lives.

Ned already knew many of the doctors and nurses, but Annie soon befriended hospital personnel as well and became a welcome fixture. Her sartorial choice was scrubs and t-shirts; she ate hospital food and, in theory, slept in a bed next to Hank's crib. In reality, and against the rules, she scooped her son out of his cage to nestle with her each night, while hospital personnel looked the other way, knowing, as she did, that this was not a time for a very sick boy to sleep alone. Monitoring devices showed that these hours with his mother stabilized his heart rate, allowing his body to rest and repair. A mother's instinct trumped medical protocol.

Ned's balancing act became even more complex. He maintained his schedule, in and out of the operating room both day and night, but he also managed to spend a great deal of time with Hank. He plugged visits into every spare minute and, when possible, took family leave time to be with him. Superman with superpowers, he somehow created extra hours in each day by seeming to be in several places at once. And, of course, he never complained because superheroes do what needs to be done in order to save humanity, or in this case, his son and family.

Not wanting to lose daily touch with Georgia, Annie, and Ned when he was able, came home every evening at 6:00 for dinner and a chance to give their daughter some semblance of normal family life. They used the time to read stories and tuck Georgia into bed, catch up with each other and relax into this other world of ordinary habits before returning to the hospital.

Bruce and Paula, Annie's parents, didn't have my level of discretionary time, but they took off as many days from work as possible to be with their daughter and her family. The agony of distance can be greater than the challenge of presence, so I can only imagine how deeply they wanted to be with the family and know how hard they tried to make it happen whenever possible.

After weeks of worry from afar, they drove down from Idaho for a long Thanksgiving weekend. While they were there, I returned home and, after they left, George, Annie's brother, moved into the house to provide whatever support he could manage while balancing a full load of graduate classes. This amazing man had already devoted every spare hour to providing aid in countless ways, many of them under the radar, but immensely important to the smooth functioning of a family in crisis. He ran errands, did minor maintenance around the house, played silly games with the kids and wore a big smile throughout. With an uncanny sense of how to be in the right place at the right time, George filled in gaps with a generosity of spirit that belied the impact on his academic life.

Annie's parents came back for Christmas and I returned in early January, prepared once again to stay as long as necessary, grateful for the opportunity to be a small player in this very large drama unfolding in unknown directions with an open-ended timeline. Although it had felt good to be home for several weeks, my mind had remained in Salt Lake City. I talked with either Annie or Ned almost every day, thought of little else but Hank and his struggling family, and tried to summon some sense of delight in the holiday, but celebration was out of the question.

The definition of "home" began to have the same fuzzy borders that many of our other habits and markers had developed. None of us quite knew where it was any more, as it changed, from geography to concept, from absolute to variable, according to the situation. I now more or less lived in Salt Lake City, Annie and Ned pretty much lived in the hospital and others lived in their frustration at not being able to do more for this beleaguered family. We all dwelled in a survival state, with food, sleep and the quest for some semblance of emotional stability our only requirements.

Since we had long ago opened to whatever religious practice came our way, it didn't seem the least bit strange to have Tibetan prayer flags strung around Hank's room while Ned's and Annie's neighbors and good friends, Spencer and Dan, came in to offer a Mormon prayer. We loved knowing a Mennonite community in Kansas, a Lutheran church in Minnesota, and a friend who went to mass every day at St. Patrick's Cathedral in New York City represented many others who were praying hard for Hank. It was extraordinarily comforting to welcome these good intentions and great spiritual energy, regardless of the belief system each represented. This was a time for complete ecumenism; everything about it felt right and kept all of us safe.

We're not sure how it happened, or who organized it (although this was obviously the work of neighbors and friends), but we had received word shortly after Hank entered the hospital that meals would be delivered to our door twice a week for as long as we needed them. Full, delicious repasts, tucked into baskets or boxes, miraculously showed up just when we didn't have another ounce of energy to pull something together. These meals were usually preceded by phone calls saying when they would arrive, but occasionally they just appeared—no donor identification, no chat at the door. Gifts of flowers, bath salts, books and toys also turned up on the front porch. We came to understand that, although most came from preschool or doctor friends, some reflected the generosity of strangers, mostly Mormons, who simply saw a need and met it in the best way possible. Once again, this neighborhood, where few really knew the outsiders, practiced what their religion preached, requiring no thanks, no recognition—only doing what seemed right, with anonymity showing authenticity.

Annie, eyes on the horizon, did two amazing things during this time: not only was she Hank's nurse/support system/cheerleader, but she also got pregnant. And she met both situations with characteristic equanimity, still facing the days ahead with the expectation that everything would come out all right, the only option she could imagine. Her pregnancy was a deliberate decision by the young parents, one meant to grow their family if the unthinkable happened. We were all astonished that she would deliberately accept another major challenge, but she was determined and nothing would change her mind.

In contrast to the other scenario unfolding in the halls of medicine, three-year-old Georgia's two mornings in preschool gave me small breaks while leaving plenty of time for the two of us to have great fun together. We read endless books, created art projects, went to the library and museums, told each other stories and made frequent trips to the hospital to check in with Mom or Dad and Hank. Georgia needed to be part of his life without being overwhelmed, so these small visits were perfect.

"Hank, look what I brought you!" She might produce a flower, or dead bug, or rock or other random item that she thought her brother might like. "This is a picture I drew of you holding a snake!" "This rock is ten gazillion years old!" "I found the bug lying on his back with his feet sticking up in the air!" He rarely responded verbally, but his eyes lit up when she came into the room and the two of them played until he became tired—usually within ten or fifteen minutes. Those few times were usually the highlight of his day.

Whenever Georgia met someone new—a librarian, store clerk, waitress, mail carrier or in any other random encounter—she delivered the following speech, with its content never varying: "Do you know my brother Hank? He's in the 'hosipul' because his heart doesn't work. But he's going to be all right. Mommy and Daddy are there with him, so I know he's going to be all right." Some people just smiled in a confused sort of way. But most picked up on her earnestness and knew exactly how to reply to a little girl who needed affirmation from strangers in order to process the profusion of frightening events. "I'm sure he will be just fine," they usually replied with as much enthusiasm as they could muster, whereupon Georgia brightened into their promise, pleased that the circle of supporters had just grown a little larger.

One evening, Annie returned to Hank's room at 8:00 to find one of their favorite nurses with her son. This burly guy with a beard and ponytail held Hank on his knee while they both watched "Bridge to Terabithia" on TV. Hank wasn't tuned in to the story line, but tears ran down the nurse's cheeks. What better place than in the safety of a movie to put the emotions that assault medical personnel in a children's hospital? This level of compassion showed up in countless ways among the staff throughout Hank's stay and became even more overt as, regardless of intention, he slowly wriggled into their hearts.

Hank's condition continued to deteriorate as weeks turned into months. Because the PICU bred a hotbed of germs, all of which were looking for vulnerable hosts, he was moved to the surgical recovery unit. Always the trooper, he took up residence in his new room and adapted to this environment as though crossing it off his to-do list.

When he wasn't resting in someone's arms, Hank crawled down onto a floor mat to examine the ever-shifting variety of toys that kept showing up. He took things apart and tried to put them together, played little xylophones, flutes, drums and other music-makers and looked at books. Because he still required regular monitoring, a revolving door of medical personnel stopped by, either to check on their favorite patient or just to chat with his mom or dad. Every nurse, technician and doctor brought a sweet and gentle spirit into the room, delivering an energy boost to both patient and family. These were his friends and, on some level, his playmates. Although this hospital was filled with sick kids, there was no interaction among them. An infection could have put any of them in great danger, so everyone scrubbed up before entering rooms and then used hand sanitizer to boot. Anyone with a sniffle appeared in a mask, a scenario that didn't faze Hank.

He was masked as well for occasional adventures into the great world beyond his room. An IV pole rolled alongside him under the control of whatever adult accompanied his exploration. On these forays, which always followed the same path and pattern, his practice was to stop in front of each familiar nurse, doctor or technician. He looked up with those huge eyes, waited for acknowledgement and a pat on the head, made no sound, and then suddenly turned and marched on, bound for his next small destination. The mask disallowed facial expression, so we never knew whether he was smiling in response to these individual encounters—like a Halloween caller who takes his candy and disappears into the night.

Hank always stopped to examine the fish painted on the wall and he often pushed a wooden lawnmower/popper or a large plastic car that he had carefully loaded with toys. Sometimes he went to a door and tried to open it. These attempts to rejoin the world were the most heart-rending moments of all.

Occasionally he needed to just stop and rest, but then he trudged on in his slow, methodical way. When he was just too tired to continue, he got a ride back in the arms of his companion. The entire journey was probably never more than sixty or seventy feet, but they were miles to him and left him exhausted. However, his parents insisted that he get out of that small room and into the greater world of the hallway, both for physical and neurological stimulation. Even when he didn't feel like it, he forced himself to do it, desperate for any change in routine.

In the greater picture, it was a small annoyance, but Annie, of course, had morning sickness, although she never mentioned it. This discomfort simply became part of her surreal existence. Scrubs, with their large, drawstring waists, now provided perfect sartorial support for her expanding middle. Her body grew as her son struggled unsuccessfully to reach even the lowest weight percentile on the doctor's chart.

We weren't deeply tuned into the fact that Hank didn't talk much. He seemed to understand what was being said, but, due to the tube in his throat and other factors, he couldn't speak without some discomfort, so he remained mostly silent. His needs were met, he wasn't in the company of other babbling kids, and, I'm guessing, speaking took more effort than he could muster at that point. We didn't really expect him to experiment with sounds and words and didn't think it strange that he wasn't engaged in vocal practice. Actually, we weren't too sure about his cognitive state, but his lack of interest in talking was the least of our worries at this point, and his body language spoke all we needed to know.

The days and weeks blurred together, but on one afternoon the hospital buzzed with unusual excitement. Members of the city's professional basketball team, the Utah Jazz, accompanied by their mascot, a man in a very hairy bear costume, were coming to visit the patients. What more could hospitalized kids want than a visit from famous athletes? At least that's what celebrity visitors and hospital personnel have always assumed. However, no one seemed to consider that seven-foot-tall men and a life-size bear might be alarming to a sick child of seventeen months whose only experience with basketball had consisted of watching small figures run around on a TV screen while sitting on his father's lap. Men and women wearing half masks on their faces were a common occurrence, but nothing prepared Hank for a bear leaping in the door, followed by very tall strangers with lots of athletic energy and little sense of the impact they might have on a toddler.

Hank was paralyzed with fear, but, accustomed now to all sorts of unexpected situations, he managed to remain respectful. Instead of gasping in alarm or diving under a blanket, he turned to his only communication tool. He blew them kisses and frantically waved bye-bye while his mother suggested that they beat a hasty retreat. Hank let out a sigh of relief, but kept a wary eye on the door in case they decided to invade again, which, thankfully, they didn't. They did, however, leave a small basketball and a teddy bear wearing a costume similar to that of the giant creature that had scared the daylights out of him. Hank demanded that the stuffed animal disappear immediately. He would never again be in the same room with Jazz Bear, or any other teddy bear for that matter.

Ned and Annie's home was so close to the hospital complex that medical evacuation helicopters buzzed overhead several times a day. Before Hank's birth, these great birds held a certain power for me as I imagined their passengers in life and death scenarios and always sent them a small blessing. But, while my grandson was waiting for a heart, their appearance took on new significance. I now found myself wondering, each time I heard their roar, whether Hank's future heart might be on board. Always pausing after this thought, I felt a bit guilty but then remembered that my hope had no connection with outcome and was just a harmless pastime.

I couldn't stop imagining a heart beating somewhere that would one day find its way into my grandson's chest. The fact that a new heart for Hank required another small soul—who was, at that very moment, running, laughing and playing—to leave the world was a philosophical rumination far too profound for my brain. But it repeatedly wound through my thoughts. How is it possible to wish for an event that would bring such loss on one end and such joy on the other?

Hank's name was on a list that included virtually all patients in the western states. At any given time, more than 3,000 people await hearts in the United States, but only around 2,000 to 2,500 donors are found each year. Not only are families often unwilling to offer this gift, but, even if they make that choice, the heart may not be a candidate for a variety of reasons. Transplants are awarded priority by time on a wait list, but other factors also enter into the decision. These include severity of the recipient's illness, distance between the donor and transplant hospitals and the family's ability to provide necessary post-surgical support. But the measure, without which the others don't matter, is the degree of match. This complex stew of numbers and factors helps make the decision when the donor heart becomes available.

Although I, and Hank's greater circle, grew into this under-standing at different rates, we all ultimately arrived at a place I like to call "the great letting go," not of Hank himself but of our expectations about how things should look. As Joseph Campbell said, "If you want to make God laugh, tell Him your plans." Life has a habit of slapping assumptions around, and, looking back, these were truly our times of great learning. During the months of waiting, time became a Dali clock, melting its inconstancy into our expectations, repeatedly speeding or slowing until we just gave up and worked to separate ourselves from its consequences. Our success with this intention was erratic, but as the icy weather outside served as a metaphor for our struggles, attempts at detachment became feeble at best. Quiet despair began to lurk in the corners.

Few of us ever knew the date; we often had to stop and think a moment to name the day of the week. We grabbed handfuls of nuts or whatever snack was handy rather than worrying about balanced meals. Conversations consisted almost solely of updates on Hank's condition. He hadn't eaten more than a few Cheerios all day. He had thrown up what he had eaten. The feeding tube was inadequate. He had lost weight. We didn't speculate on where this was going because we had lost the ability to move beyond the time and space of that moment. We didn't read books, rarely talked to friends on the phone. We didn't remember to pick up emails or imagine being elsewhere, doing something other than waiting and watching.

Hank had been in the hospital since early November. By mid-January, things looked increasingly grim. His only real form of nourishment came through the feeding tube, a desperate attempt to get something into his system that might maintain his fragile frame. At eighteen months, he hadn't gained an ounce since entering the hospital, weighing only eighteen pounds and presenting more bones than flesh. Pulmonary pressures climbed, a sign that his lungs weren't functioning adequately. He couldn't swallow anything without vomiting. Even water couldn't stay down. Frustrated and desperate, he repeatedly tried to pull out the NG (nasogastric) tube that put a bit of nourishment directly into his stomach. In a last ditch effort, the doctors replaced it with a NJ (naso-jejunal) tube that went directly into his small intestine, hoping this one would stay planted. He was completely miserable, very weak and extremely compromised. His systems, inadequately supported by blood flow, were shutting down and the doctors had no other treatment options. Their faces grew increasingly grave as they dropped by to examine Hank and consult his chart, and finally, with greatest tact, they let Ned and Annie know that, if this trend continued, he would possibly be removed from the transplant list. A committee would be meeting soon to make this decision. With a body so frail, his chances of surviving surgery were becoming almost negligible, and the donor heart that might keep another child alive would be wasted if his body couldn't accept it. Ned tried without success to be philosophical and dispassionate, but Annie couldn't even process the words. She still believed strongly that something amazing waited just around the corner.

I have no idea how Ned and Annie shared their feelings about this diminishment with each other, or whether they even dared put them into words, but one evening Annie and I finally talked, carefully and honestly, about this reality. We tried to imagine what was coming—but found it an exercise in impossibility. For so long we had maintained the level of numb equanimity that had carried us through each gray and dismal winter day. Now, looking back, I realize we simply couldn't process this descent into hopelessness. We were, without saying it, in the process of slow surrender. With no other place to turn, we decided to try to re-energize the prayer/energy burst that had brought us so much comfort a few months earlier. I called my sister, Melinda, asking her to put out the word that we needed help and we needed it now, hoping that metaphorical knees might hit the floor again. It was all we could do, and it was everything.

THREE

"A night is but small breath and little pause,
To answer matters of this consequence."

William Shakespeare

∞

THE FOLLOWING EVENING, Annie and I once again tried to muster a sliver of optimism as we chatted over dinner, but hope was as fleeting as smoke in a hurricane. She tucked Georgia into bed and left for the hospital. Five minutes later, the phone rang and a man identifying himself as Doctor Norlin asked for Annie. When told she had just left, he asked for Ned. "Is everything all right?" I asked.

"Oh, yes!" he assured me. I knew immediately. My first impulse was to call Annie, but I decided to wait. It would take fifteen minutes for her to drive, park, talk to the doctor and call me. I paced, looked at my watch, looked at the phone, checked my watch again. Exactly fifteen minutes later, the phone rang and a sobbing Annie announced, "Hank's getting a heart! It's coming from California! It's happening! Bring Georgia to the hospital! It's happening tonight!"

Ned, meanwhile, was at a restaurant dinner for prospective residents when his phone rang. "Oh, my gosh! I'm on my way!" he shouted. Then, to his fellow residents, "I gotta go! I gotta go right now!" They, without needing to ask, leaped to their feet and hugged him as the bewildered candidates watched in astonishment. I'm sure they could have guessed for the rest of the evening and not come close to imagining the scenario that was about to unfold. In a few seconds,

Ned sprinted from the restaurant and sped toward the event he had feared would never happen.

I called my daughter, Bryn, and my husband, Dave, then the neighbors and friends who were all a huge part of Team Hank. A quick group email to the hundred or so people on the "must notify" list and calls to a few other close relatives began the communication process. I imagined telephone lines and emails blazing through the night as the network was put on high alert, gathering in a holy circle around this little boy and his stunned family

"I want you to let me know, whatever time it is, when the new heart is in place," my sister insisted. "But it will be in the middle of the night," I said. "No problem," she replied. "Do it!" She would then call her adult children, who would be waiting for word. Other relatives and friends also requested instant communication, a promise I wasn't sure I could keep.

My other son, Bridge, was at a workshop retreat a thousand miles away in the mountains of Georgia, and was not to be disturbed, but I had asked for an emergency number and was able to call the caretaker. "I can't take messages unless it's an emergency," the man announced in an irritated voice.

"Please tell him his nephew will get a new heart tonight," I shouted. "He's having a transplant!"

A few seconds of silence. "Oh yes, ma'am, I'll get word to him right away," the man gasped. "And I'll be praying for that little boy." Bridge called a few minutes later, choking his words, wishing desperately he could be standing with us by Hank's side.

Georgia had no idea what was really happening but she knew it was very exciting. She began to spin around, singing, "Hank's getting a heart! Hank's getting a heart!" We scurried through the house, almost running into each other as we packed a bag for a quickly scheduled overnight with her next-door friend, Emma, and then dashed to the hospital. Time wasn't really of the essence, but it seemed critical that we get there as soon as possible.

Georgia and I arrived in Room 3085 to find it buzzing with people and cacophony, not unlike a New Year's Eve party as midnight approaches. Doctors, nurses and other personnel had converged from all over the hospital to offer congratulations to Ned and Annie, while assuring Hank that all would go well and he was going to be all right. There were no streamers or confetti, but in my mind the room was wild with color. Hugs, laughter and conversation swirled around the parents and a very confused child. And of course, Georgia loved the party, laughing and jumping around the room, eager to join the celebration. No one bothered to stay quiet. This level of festivity in anticipation of life-threatening surgery was a bit difficult for me to fully appreciate, but I joined in the festivities in a somewhat subdued way.

Friends slowly drifted out, reluctant to say good-bye and sobered now to what lay ahead. I whisked Georgia to her friend's house to stay the night and sped back to Hank's hospital room where I found Ned, Annie, and her brother, George, in a more tempered state, trying to prepare for whatever the night would bring. It was 9:00. Hank was to leave for surgery at 11:00. He slept soundly in his mother's arms as his parents whispered above.

Just as things calmed down, a great dervish of a priest, called by Ned from the foxhole of desperation, flew in the door to do his magic. He whirled around the room, distributing old-fashioned "holy cards" with pictures of saints. We grabbed them as though they were hand-delivered from heaven and printed with magic ink. The priest finally settled down and spoke softly to Hank, now awake, and then began to read obscure incantations over this puzzled child while we watched from afar, unsure of what might be happening. Trying without success to sense a heavenly light descending, we just hoped the priest would leave soon. By the time he backed out the door, we felt sanctified and relieved. All bases had been covered.

As the room filled with silence, reality appeared. In two hours, the little boy who looked at us with wide eyes and complete trust would be wheeled into the inner sanctum where medicine's most sacred ceremonies are performed. His tiny chest would be invaded, the tattered organ that commands all others would be removed and a gift of ineffable value would be stitched into its place. A family was saying good-bye a half continent away; we were saying good-bye to the rhythm that had marked our lives for eighteen months, and, quite possibly, inconceivably, we were saying good-bye to Hank. The train was leaving and we would hold on by our fingernails as it streaked full-throttle ahead.

Nurses tiptoed in to prepare the patient, and then George and I left the parents in the privacy of that quiet, dark room. I found a desk in the hallway and wrote in my journal:

Dearest Hank:

On this evening when time has stopped and we hardly dare breathe, all wait. You sit like a Buddha in the midst of a whirlwind, amazingly peaceful, as though you know the time you've so long expected has come at last. Our emotions range from a terrified excitement to a frozen calm, as we try to process the knowledge that new life will soon fly through this night sky in a small container so filled with complexity that words can't possibly find a place to rest within its many implications.

A very young person is about to depart the world under circumstances we'll never know, leaving behind a tiny gift for a stranger. I try to comprehend that the child whose heart is about to come to you is at this moment still alive and that his or her family is mourning as we rejoice. I send them a silent blessing with the hope that their generosity will bring some small measure of comfort during this terrible time. I also imagine the private jet winging toward California to retrieve its precious cargo—the very essence of life carried like crown jewels, although far more valuable.

You rest now in the company of only your parents, all preparations accomplished—blood drawn, drugs administered, bathed like a gladiator about to enter the arena. Throughout this time you watch, eyes moving from face to face, as though seeking confirmation of something you already know. You are telling us not to worry. You seem to remember your assignment, facing it without fear. The time has arrived.

Because transplant surgeries can be scheduled, they are almost always performed during the night, when no other procedures can get in the way. Midnight, with its attendant emotional charge, is the preferred hour. At 11:20, the transport team arrived in his room and Hank was moved from his mother's arms to a rolling crib where he opened his eyes, sat up and remained in that position on his trip to surgery. During the elevator ride, as we squeezed around his crib, he looked at each of us with long gazes held for several seconds—no complaints, no fear, only peaceful resignation. We each managed small smiles as we accompanied him on the winding path to this unimaginable destination, wondering how we would say good-bye.

51

Long, deserted corridors echoed our passage at that hour approaching midnight, with no other sounds to be heard. Around the last corner stood a group of people in scrubs and caps—surgeons, anesthesiologists, cardiologists, nurses, intensivists, perfusionists— awaiting this momentous event, one unlike any other surgery. They spoke softly to us, excited and ready for their turn. It was time for a final farewell. I kissed my grandson quickly and wished him well, small tears coming despite my best efforts and intentions. His Mom and Dad, those paragons of stoicism, smiled and spoke to him once again of their love, kissed and hugged him for what could have been the last time and then watched dry-eyed as he was wheeled down the corridor. Although many children would cry and reach out for their parents, Hank remained still and silent, looking back at them with pure trust. He might have been blowing kisses, but perhaps he was looking ahead as he left on his magnificent journey.

Ned, Annie, George and I adjourned to the nearby waiting room, unsure of a timeline or sequence of events, and, after a while, Annie and I made nests on the floor from flannel sheets that had been stacked in the corner. Ned paced. George sat in a chair, staring into space. No one else was in the room or corridor and the hospital was absolutely silent, the perfect setting for contemplation as we took up our long vigil. Nodding off was virtually impossible. I went back and forth from floor to chair, tried to read, wrote in my journal, closed my eyes, thought I should pray but found it impossible to gather my thoughts into straight lines. Instead, I imagined myself with Hank, stroking his arm, assuring him that everything would be all right. Each of us—Annie, Ned, George and I—wrapped ourselves in the personal cocoon we required for comfort. Far beyond conversation, we communed by being in each other's presence and exchanging glances and wary smiles every once in a while.

When I call up those hours, I most remember whiteness—walls, blankets, minds, emotions—all without color, everything indistinct. I couldn't summon coherence or sequence; expectation had yielded to surrender of control. I felt no fear, only numbness, as we simply waited for life, or its opposite, to play out.

What happened next provided a sudden focus for our attention—an unwelcome, astonishing connection with Hank. We heard his heart beat. An accidental flip of a switch broadcast every sound from the operating room throughout our wing of the hospital. Beneath mumbled conversation, a rhythmic beat throbbed. Hank was connecting with us in the most elemental code. Although I was somewhat comforted by this anomaly, Annie sat up from her nest on the floor and pleaded, "Make it stop! Get someone to turn it off!"

Ned had gone for a walk, so I streaked through the hallways, looking for someone, anyone, to bring quiet back to our space. But the corridors, nursing stations, even the rooms in our wing were completely deserted. I finally dashed down to the first-floor cafeteria, thinking someone might know how to address this bizarre turn of events. Rushing up to a nurse carrying a tray, I quickly explained the situation and location. She looked at me in horror and we both set off at a fast clip for the elevators. In a strange coincidence, she was the only duty nurse for the surgical wing on that night; I had found the perfect person. We rode up to the third floor, she disappeared around a corner, and within a minute silence returned. Not long after, she entered our waiting room, arms loaded with warm flannel sheets, and offered an apology for the freakish circumstance no one could explain. It had been unnerving, but also astonishing to hear Hank's steady rhythm speak to us—a last, strange communication to a waiting family several long corridors away who could think of nothing but that small cadence reaching out to us.

When a heart becomes available, the events surrounding it are organized with Swiss-watch precision, and every detail is under tight control. The recipient family must be within immediate reach, a condition to which all listed families agree—no trips out of town, no deviation from expectation or the entire process is scratched. If everything matches up, a private jet, containing a surgeon and support team, streaks to its destination. The donor heart, which has continued beating by artificial means after its owner has left earthly bonds, is injected with potassium chloride to stop its pulse. It is then, to use the unfortunate medical term, "harvested" by the visiting team. The heart is placed in a "cold box," where the temperature is regulated to maintain viability.

By this means, Hank's new heart began its wild journey, packed in ice and tucked into a virtual picnic cooler, an inelegant transfer device for such powerful contents but the only process known to the medical community at that time. The organ's viability had begun deteriorating right after removal and would continue to do so for up to six hours, at which point it would no longer be usable. Because each moment was precious and each action part of a tightly orchestrated survival drama, time was of the utmost essence. The surgeon, support team and precious cooler were rushed by ambulance through dark streets accompanied by wailing sirens. Upon arriving at the airport with special clearance, the vehicle drove directly to the waiting small plane, where passengers and cargo were quickly secured before the craft took off through the night on its mission of mercy, with the destination several hundred miles away.

1:10 a.m. The first call comes to the waiting room. "The plane has landed; estimated time of arrival is 20 minutes." The ambulance drives at warp speed through the sleeping streets of Salt Lake City, sirens once again screaming. In the operating room at Primary Children's Hospital, a median sternotomy has been performed, the pericardium opened and great vessels dissected. Hank is attached to a cardiopulmonary bypass machine as all wait for the precious package.

1:40 a.m. We receive a call saying the heart has arrived in the operating room; the transplant is beginning. We look at each other, wordless, and sink even more deeply into the very small and private place each of us now occupies. I try not to imagine him lying on the table, chest wide open, completely vulnerable. Nothing else fills my mind's eye, and so I yield to that connection, imagining myself standing by his side, holding his hand.

Is there a place on the other side of the atmosphere already described? We are there, having now entered a space so surreal that nothing even looks familiar in the small warren where we try to capture immensity. We simply exist, breathe in and out, float slightly outside our bodies and let go of everything. Time is only a theory; I look at the clock every few minutes but can't process its message. Imagination flares and dims, unable to capture the ephemeral.

My dearest Hank,

Where are you now? Winging your way around an unknown sky? Seeing yourself from above the table? Running fast and free? Watching us? Will you come back, and, if so, what will you carry from your months in a foreign land and your hours in a space beyond all known borders?

Most of us try to imagine a future that surpasses our ability to anticipate, but Ned's mind is in the operating room, observing a surgery in which he has participated many times. He sees each step, knows the timing and imagines every possible departure from expectation. His son's frayed heart will be removed by transecting great vessels and part of the left atrium. The pulmonary veins, and a circle of the atrium containing them, will remain. The donor heart will be trimmed to fit into this space and the great vessels sutured into place. A thousand things can go wrong and he knows about each of them. He stares at the phone, willing it to yield the only words he can bear to hear.

3:10 a.m. The phone brings us to high alert. All hearts pound. This is the moment that will change our world forever, the one we've long anticipated with both terror and the smallest glimmer of hope. We can't bear to look at each other so watch Ned closely. He picks up the receiver before he has a chance to fear the news. The words are good, very good. The new heart has found a home and is beating with vigor. Hank's body is reacting just as the doctors had hoped, with all systems reviving. I imagine blood pumping into his lungs, through his liver, kidneys, digestive system and all the way to his little fingers and toes. He is turning pink all over. He is coming back to life.

The new heart has received some electrical stimulation, but the magic of a spontaneous beat that continues in a different body remains the stuff of mystery. The bypass support is removed and the surgical team watches in wonder as the transplanted organ shivers back to life and finds its pace after spending several inert hours on ice. A doctor will explain that it's a self-generated stimulus that comes from the sinoatrial, or SA, node, the heart's internal pacemaker. It's known as the cardiac conduction system, a fiber bundle that conveys a bio-electrical signal to and from the heart. In thirty minutes, the rhythm of Hank's heart has stabilized enough to remove the bypass mechanism. I care little for the science or the theory, preferring to think of it only as a pure, unadulterated miracle.

There are no tears or high fives, but we manage weak smiles. This is only the beginning and celebration is not in the program, although quiet relief engulfs us all. As surgeons close the gaping incision, we make calls to people who lie awake around the country, waiting to hear. Talking quietly among ourselves now, we begin to process the fact that life is continuing, that Hank has survived the surgery. The days ahead can't even be imagined, but none of that matters; our boy is alive and the heart is pumping with absolute glee.

I send a blessing from my own heart to the California family who returned home this night to an empty crib. I press their pain next to our gratitude in a strange blend of conflicting emotions that simply can't find a place to rest. With no other response available, I hold them in the light and send waves of peace and comfort over the miles, hoping they'll feel some small measure of our gratitude, an imperfect word to describe the rapture of hope, the passion of thankfulness that now glows in our deepest, most wordless places.

When Dr. Hawkins, the transplant surgeon, comes to report, we gather his words with care and place them in a memory basket for later retrieval and transmission. Those of us without a medical background have nothing but these discrete bits of information from which to weave a new truth. We want to make sure we have the straight story so we listen with intense concentration: "Hank's heart was, to put it bluntly, a disaster. It had to work so hard that it was greatly enlarged, but the new heart is a normal size, much smaller than his, so drainage tubes will release any fluids that build up in the extra space left behind. To tell you the truth, the new heart came just in time; he couldn't have lasted much longer. He's a strong little guy. I think he will be fine, but it will be a tough road for all of you."

Later that night, Ned, driven by both curiosity and a need for a different kind of closure, slipped into the pathology lab with a strange request. He wanted to examine the heart that had been removed from a little boy a few hours earlier. Against rules and against protocol, the person on duty decided to make an exception, and within a few minutes, my son was holding his son's heart in his hand. He found it profoundly damaged—the left ventricle spongy, with porous walls—and was amazed that this child had managed to summon the strength of spirit to survive with such a deeply flawed machine in control of his body. In its effort to pump, it had grown to the size of a small orange, while its replacement was not much bigger than a walnut, thus leaving the space referred to by the surgeon. This pocket would gradually fill in, but would require monitoring and draining as the body adjusted itself around the intruder. Hank's heart would be used for research, his case having already appeared in several cardiology review publications.

George and I dragged home around 6:00 a.m., feeling neither elation nor despair but only a continuing sense of suspension, the kind of empty space that surrounds a sleepless night and a tenuous future. Ned and Annie were allowed into the inner sanctum of Intensive Care to look at, and maybe touch the hand of, their son. Now pink of cheek, he nonetheless looked vulnerable on a ventilator, his entire chest swathed in a thick, white bandage and lines once again radiating out to machines. His new heart spoke to a cadre of scurrying medical personnel in beeps and lines on a screen, an arcane but welcome communication. Although this would be impossible for several days, his parents ached to hold him close, but Ned's exhaustion knew no descriptors and, on top of dealing with the fatigue of pregnancy, Annie was carrying an incipient illness that had been building for days. Knowing Hank wasn't aware of their presence, they at last pulled themselves away and limped home to bed.

An hour of fitful sleep for me was interrupted by several phone calls in immediate response to the quick email I had sent upon returning to the house. My sister, Kate, dashed out the door to tell the grocery store clerk, mail carrier and librarian, along with other friends, the amazing news. My friend called her mother in Atlanta, who had never met Hank but immediately burst into tears. Relatives called or emailed to say they were sending all good thoughts our way. I imagined supporters contacting friends throughout the country and remembered once again that this cast was comprised of hundreds.

I retrieved Georgia from Emma's house and shared the news. "Guess what? Hank has a brand new heart and now he's going to feel so much better! He has to stay in the hospital a while longer, but then he'll be home to stay!"

"Will Mommy and Daddy come home, too?" she ventured hopefully. "Will we all sleep in the same house? All of the time? From now on?" She didn't quite believe my affirmative answers, but although I couldn't guarantee the truth of my promises, it felt very good to offer her this gift at long last.

Annie, finally released from her need to maintain constant watch over Hank, virtually collapsed into a full-blown state of respiratory onslaught. With heightened flu symptoms attacking a body that had been compromised and challenged for so long, her defenses were completely exhausted. She could only stumble into bed, where she stayed for twenty-four hours, declining all food and connection with the outside world. Fortunately, her parents arrived and began helping out in every way possible, providing Annie with the safety and nurturing available only from her own mother and father. We all gathered tightly and continued to live from hour to hour, delighted to share this time with each other.

FOUR

"My long sickness
Of health and living now begins to mend..."

William Shakespeare

THE DETACHED SENSATION CONTINUED THROUGH THAT DAY, with sleep not returning until evening. Ned and I went back to the hospital a few hours later, eager to see the warrior returned from battle with a great glory scar. Masked, gowned and gloved, we tiptoed into a room that closely resembled command central for a presidential medical procedure. Nurses in constant attention; beeps, bubbles, whistles and clicks from a bank of machines as background rhythm; and constant vigilance from an ever-changing cohort of cardiac experts set a surreal scene. Finding Hank with a huge clump of bandage on his chest, a respirator and four drainage tubes along with other lines was not unexpected but still shocking in its intensity. He was, of course, deeply sedated, a state in which he would be maintained for most of the next few days.

I couldn't leave, couldn't let go, as though watching closely might somehow keep him safer. But I also lingered because I was fascinated with the machinations surrounding this tiny patient and wanted to observe every response protocol in great detail. Highly specialized nurses continuously bustled around and hovered over him. I listened carefully as they shared their observations with each other and with the doctors, who closely relied on them for both information and opinions.

We were stunned to hear that Hank's surgeon, who dropped by after spending the night crafting my grandson's new life, was on his way to another major surgery. Completely sleep-deprived and barely able to string words together, he was nonetheless about to undertake another godlike act while under the beck and call of Morpheus. My only thought was gratitude that the next patient wasn't Hank. I also wondered about this kind of scheduling, but assumed this was the exception more than rule and that he, like most people in positions of great responsibility, had learned to soldier through a challenge that would flatten the rest of us for days.

Under the influence of multiple potions that represent western medicine at its finest, Hank's heart gradually made uneasy peace with his body. Massive doses of steroids and immunosuppressants, along with a host of other concoctions, spoke a language his systems understood.

His extubation (removal of the breathing tube) a few hours later was short-lived, as Hank simply couldn't suck in enough air, one of many frightening responses that appeared during the next few days. It was determined that his throat was swollen from hours of intubation and that a smaller tube would need to be inserted until he could breathe independently. But good news arrived in the form of something called an ejection fraction, a measure of the pumping strength in his left ventricle. We had followed this number faithfully for several months, slightly relieved when it climbed to the mid-twenties, uneasy when it fell lower. The new heart measured seventy. His pulmonary function, in the high and dangerous nineties two days earlier, now showed up at a delightful ten, another positive sign of a strong heart. Faith is a tenuous but necessary quality during times like these, and we held it with caution.

Annie, however, exuded confidence from every pore. After coming back from her collapsing illness, one of her first acts was to order a new wardrobe for Hank from her favorite children's catalog. This child, whose sartorial expression had been limited to a diaper and t-shirt for the past several months, was about to re-enter the greater world, and she would be ready. Her conviction inspired our own, and we began to imagine the possibility that Hank might eventually become a participant on a wider stage, something we hadn't dared consider.

The next day, Hank began to twitch and then to thrash, undoubtedly from pain but also as he tried to escape confinement. His nurse had no choice. She tied his hands to the railing so he couldn't pull out any tubes—a sight that broke our hearts. But good news trumped bad—he was gradually returning to the world. With the removal of two drainage tubes, one so large that a stitch was required to close the exit area, only one remained in his chest. He had stabilized for the moment but his condition remained tenuous and still required constant monitoring. Annie ached to hold her child, to feel his body against her own, but it wasn't quite time yet. So she stroked his arm, his head, his feet, talked to him and waited.

Hank still slept on the third day, but he was without restraints when we visited in the morning and seemed much more peaceful. His breathing tube was taken out in the afternoon and, to everyone's relief, he managed well on his own, another huge step toward recovery. Best of all, when I returned that afternoon, he was nestled in his mother's grateful arms, still groggy and semi-conscious but undoubtedly feeling the comfort of her presence. Tubes stretched from his body to various machines, but Annie was skilled in maneuvering around these fetters. She was radiant; he was pink but puffy from steroids and fluid retention. But he was absolutely beautiful from head to toe. Her eyes drank him in, scanning every inch, whispering, cooing, sighing, softly laughing. Her boy slept in her arms and life was as good as it could get. Ned stood by her side, waiting to take a turn.

On the fourth day, Hank gifted us by opening his eyes slightly, but best of all, he whispered "Mama." A few minutes later, however, he began to spit up great quantities of what appeared to be old blood, either a holdover from intubation or a steroid reaction. A red and puffy face and swollen knee caused temporary concern until doctors tied those symptoms to a negative sulfa response. Each day, almost each hour, brought a new and unexpected symptom, and we who knew nothing of what was going on, or what to expect, continued to teeter. We found ourselves tiptoeing and whispering, afraid to believe everything would eventually resolve itself. It was all so complex, so mysterious and even the doctors seemed to be guessing more than our comfort level could allow.

On day five, Hank continued to have problems holding anything in his stomach, a situation now attributed to the effects of two different morphine doses—one to ease the pain of removing the last, large drainage tube and the other to address agitation. On the sixth day, Annie and I arrived at the hospital to find Hank sitting up in his crib, eyes wide open and bearing the discomfort of a complicated line removal with a stoic courage characteristic of him. Ned, who had been there for several hours, watched the bumbled procedure with increasing annoyance. When the nurse, for some reason, was unable to complete the procedure, Ned, unable to contain his frustration, stepped in and did the job himself, another departure from protocol, but necessary to his son's comfort. Hank later had an echocardiogram, was removed from some medications and pronounced sufficiently stable to leave the Pediatric Intensive Care Unit.

On the seventh day, he began to vomit, but doctors soon discovered the possible cause of this response—the nasogastric tube was curled around in Hank's tummy. This was promptly addressed and he soon felt better. He ate part of a popsicle and a bite or two of jello, a magnificent accomplishment, even if those two substances were from a category unrelated to food. And on the eighth day, Hank smiled, his first emotional response, and one so long awaited. He also gulped Cheerios and displayed other small, but unmistakable signs of a return to our world. He continued to be more observer than participant, still fixing his gaze on everyone and rarely talking, but he was definitely returning. He also became fussier, probably resulting more from frustration than discomfort. He walked six steps, his first attempt at ambulation, but stayed fretful, didn't sleep much and became hypersensitive toward visitors, perhaps expecting a poke, prod or prick.

Nine days after the transplant, Hank began showing signs of rejection. We all went into panic mode, but later learned that this is not unusual and would probably respond to medication. Cardiac transplant patients can have up to three rejection episodes during the first year, but that is no consolation—trepidation returned until he reacted favorably to a change in drug dosage. I couldn't stop thinking about the assault on his system of this ever-shifting array of chemicals, but then remembered the alternative and relaxed into this onslaught, hoping his body could later throw off the negative results while embracing the positive.

A hurried biopsy, in which a wire was threaded from his groin to his heart in order to snip a piece of tissue for analysis, brought the news that the inflammation, which is the first indicator of rejection, had diminished. Our fears slowly abated, but left their mark as we understood that they would always lurk around the edges of possibility. Throughout the recovery period the January weather remained a metaphoric mirror of our internal barometers, with snow, isolation, struggle and challenge shaping our days as we kept vigil beside Hank's crib. Highs and lows vacillated wildly, and we tried hard to simply accept each as just the way things were going to be for a while. We learned to move slowly while bobbing in unknown seas, unable to find destination. Hank was difficult, wonderful, challenged, happy, crabby, responsive and distant, vacillating like a feather in a fitful wind. Because each body reacts differently, the gurus of medicine could only experiment with medications and observe closely.

Dearest Hank:

As we see you in deep misery—steroid-puffy, in great pain, still suffering the after-effects of heavy anesthesia, we want you to understand something very important. Parents know no greater desperation than the inability to make their child's pain go away, and I as a grandparent feel powerless in seeing both my children and grandchild so compromised. I would truly trade places if I could buy you a healthy life, but this is your course, your assignment, your teaching as well as your learning, and we have to accept it with grace.

One night, Annie and I watched Hank closely as he played aimlessly on the floor. In guarded language, in case he understood, we discussed the part of him that hadn't given us much information—his brain. What did he comprehend? What had he lost? To what degree did he take in his world? He rarely spoke and gave few indicators that information was entering and sticking around. I decided to create a small test. I would give him serial instructions to see whether he could follow part or all of them. "Hank, will you please go over to the bed, reach in the paper bag, get the orange inside and give it to your Mom?" He looked at me as though I had just spoken in Chinese, looked at his mom, looked back at me, shrugged his shoulders and slowly stood up. He made his way to the bed, reached in the bag, extracted the orange and took it to his mom, all the while watching me closely as though he couldn't believe I'd made such a stupid request. When his mom rewarded his efforts with a big smile and huge hug the errand became worthwhile, but he kept glancing at me warily, as though I might next ask him to lick the floor or jump out of the window.

In mid-February, after five weeks away from home, it was time for me to return to Denver, although I had become so emotionally ensconced that it was hard to imagine Ned and Annie surviving without me. In reality, I'm sure they were looking forward to moving away from this level of dependence and welcoming the next chapter of family existence, something I understood and encouraged. So, with a major snowstorm brewing, I stopped at the hospital to say good-bye to a small patient who managed, according to his mother, to present his first smile of the day. Three weeks out of surgery, he was pale, miserable and still puffy from steroids, as his body worked hard to process a new recipe of chemical stew pouring through his system. I wanted nothing more than to move in next door and continue to be a present, though unobtrusive, helper, but it was not to be.

Nor was the hospital to remain his home away from home. After three months, its sounds, sights and routines were so engrained into all of us that the prospect of leaving had some aspects of regret. We had felt safe knowing Hank was in strong hands 24 hours a day. Nurses, doctors and staff had become friends, the rooms and hallways our neighborhood. None of us can find enough accolades for Primary Children's Hospital, with its highly skilled staff, atmosphere of loving competence and the absolute dedication of all personnel. Our family will remain ever grateful for the gift of this safe nest in the midst of our emotional maelstrom.

Hank was released from the hospital a few days after my departure, once again armed with a bag of medications and a portfolio of instructions. Determined to have a child like any other, Ned and Annie had talked about Hank's return home and planned how best to lead him back into new but familiar territory. Nothing about his first two years reflected a traditional childhood and nothing could erase the impact of his experience, but the chance to start over now presented itself as he struggled toward recovery. He would have no special privileges; he would become familiar with the "time out" corner; he would be loved but not overwhelmed with attention. These boundaries would be very difficult for parents who wanted nothing more than the privilege of meeting his every need and wish, but they knew his emotional survival depended on being treated like any other child.

The same philosophy would apply to Georgia, who would also need to shift her position upon Hank's return. She would no longer be a star but simply one of the kids. Three-year-olds don't usually grasp the finer points of a sibling relationship, so Ned and Annie wondered how she might react to the sudden presence of her brother. To say all went smoothly would be an exaggeration, but in fact Georgia once again rose to the occasion with both wisdom and brio. She assigned herself the position of her brother's entertainer-in-chief. Understanding his lack of energy and engagement, she decided to regale him with stories. "And when they came back, there she was, sound asleep in the baby bear's teeny-tiny bed. The daddy bear was gruff at first but later he was nice," she explained. Or, "When we were on the playground today, a big spaceship landed and took a bunch of the kids into the sky. But they came back later."

Within several weeks Hank was reported to be "almost like other boys," although this relative description came with rules and restrictions that would design his life for months to come. He played quietly, laughed and carefully explored his new, non-tethered environment. He hungered for discovery and was delighted with each new nook or toy or challenge. But his body was pumped with medication and he still fought fatigue and other unknown symptoms throughout each day. Was he in pain? Did his joints ache? Did his stomach boil?

Unfortunately, his appetite remained tenuous and his parents simply couldn't force him to eat. He broadened his food preferences and social habits ever so slightly and gained a bit of energy as time went by, but he was far from the level most kids manifest at this age. Could he see others romp and whoop with laughter without wanting to be like them? Did his brain make the connection between his life and theirs? Did he long to join the world or simply not consider the possibility that his days were supposed to look like those of other kids?

Annie and Ned dared to hope that life would return to their version of predictable, a condition in which other families existed, yet one that had seemed far out of their reach for so many months.

At seventeen weeks into her pregnancy, Annie bloomed like a ripe peach, not particularly surprised at the size of her bulge, but she began to wonder. Those muscles lose some of their elasticity by a third pregnancy, but she didn't remember being that size with the other two. An ultrasound verified what she had suspected. She was carrying twins. News that would launch most people into the stratosphere was met with philosophical acceptance by both Ned and Annie. They would deal with this the way they had dealt with so many other surprises during the past eighteen months—one step, one day at a time.

But then, two weeks later, she received devastating news: those identical girls had a condition known as Twin to Twin Transfusion (TTT), a situation that can arise in babies who share a placenta. In this frightening situation, one child pirates nutrients from the other—grabs more than its share of the goodies—resulting in an imbalance equally dangerous to both. Consequently, Annie would be closely monitored, with an ultrasound and stress tests to be performed three times a week until and unless the fluid levels equalized. If the trend continued, more drastic measures would be taken. She couldn't even begin to process this new turn of events, but instead concentrated on maintaining equanimity throughout each day. She would face the consequences as they unfolded and assume the best, although all signs pointed in another direction.

Dearest Hank:

When I came to see you, after several long weeks of wondering who you are and how you're navigating your new world, I found an amazing little boy, greatly changed in a short time! You're collecting data at record speed, soaking up everything in your new environment and continuing to impress us with your list of accomplishments—sleeping through the night in your own bed, eating lightly but better, working hard to acquire a broader vocabulary, taking things apart, and, of course, testing boundaries at every opportunity. It's not lost on any of us that these are the behaviors of every child your age, but watching them blossom in you for the first time has left me in awe. Welcome to the world of the ordinary, the prosaic, the predictable, a situation now so valued that I wonder why I never before noticed its brilliance.

Although Hank would remain captive to his house for several months, it was palatial compared with his former residence. He was still unable to have visitors, except those carefully screened for any small illness, even a cold. But he loved being home, the safe place. Georgia had dropped her brave face to become a three-year-old with mom at her side throughout the day. Mother and kids cooked, played silly games, laughed hysterically at small things and slowly knitted their family back together. Georgia and her brother became reacquainted on equal ground. The family allowed themselves to believe this might continue—that Hank would recover, that his heart would stop fighting with his body and that someday his health would not be at the forefront of their collective consciousness.

Though months were passing, it was still too early to let down their guard. The endless weeks held many frightening episodes with passing viruses, primarily brought from preschool by Georgia, but Hank fought them off as his attenuated immune system did yeoman's duty.

Those not directly involved almost forgot that panic must have lived just south of relative calm in the parents' minds. Each trip to the doctor brought them to the threshold of alarm as they wondered whether the news would be good or terrifying. Each small illness in the family could turn deadly. A pharmaceutical misstep could be life-threatening. It wouldn't be exaggerating to assume they lived in a constant state of mild Post Traumatic Stress Disorder. They could never escape and yet they had learned to manage this condition enough to relax, laugh and continually muse on the pure, unadulterated astonishment of lives that had unfolded so far from expectation.

Those medications that kept Hank alive also delivered a host of strange physical changes—all typical and expected but nonetheless startling. One of these was excessive hair growth, known to the doctors as hirsutism. Hank began to sprout silky hair all over his body—swirls and whorls on his back, on his arms and legs and even on his face. His eyelashes grew so long that, without a trim, they interfered with his vision. One of Annie's new jobs was to remove the growth from his eyebrows up to his hairline. Without cosmetic intercession, trips to the grocery store might have brought unwelcome comments, so maintaining a level of normal appearance became important. His hair darkened and his gums began to grow slightly over his teeth—all typical side effects of these powerful drugs, but ones that were still disconcerting as Hank metamorphosed before our eyes. Nonetheless, he remained our beautiful boy and these oddments became part of who he was, just as every other development over the previous two years had found its place in our lives.

Because Hank had no frame of reference, he still didn't know whether he felt bad, nor did we, but it was safe to assume that he spent most of his days in a state of aching fatigue and digestive distress. Of course he never complained; he thought life was supposed to feel that way. This initiated another interesting philosophical consideration: is dysfunction a burden or simply a state of being for those who have never known anything else?

In mid-March, at twenty-one weeks into her pregnancy, Annie heard the news she most feared. The twins' fluid levels were so imbalanced that the only hope of saving either was a delicate surgical procedure that was dangerous for both babies. Standing alone, this would be a crisis of huge proportions; juxtaposed against events of the past few months, it was something else to endure. This couple was about to face another life and death situation; they had no choice but to do so with as much courage as they could muster. Annie made an appointment with a clinic in Los Angeles that performed this procedure. She would fly out the following Monday, but before leaving would have one last measure of fluid levels. On that morning, with preparations in place and a brave face pasted on, she went to the doctor's office; the fluids were back in sufficient balance to preclude the need for surgery. She could unpack her bags and stitch together her frayed psyche. Another small miracle?

The fluid levels maintained an imbalanced equanimity—not uneven enough to warrant intervention, but never quite symmetrical either; one twin stayed higher, the other lower. By her 25th week, surgery was no longer a viable option, so hope and prayers were now directed toward a positive outcome. If only the twins could stay planted long enough to reach a healthy weight before entering the world, their chances would be good.

My son, Bridge, and I spent several delightful days captivated by the elegance of the ordinary as we returned to Hank's life later in the spring, rejoicing in simple moments played out on his small stage. We watched his habits of solitary play as he brought intense concentration to every task. We delighted in his many tender gestures toward each of us, his funny sense of humor and appreciation for the absurd. We melted in observing the bond that tied the family together in a slow dance of love.

A warm day took us to the park, where Hank watched every kid very carefully, noting play options and social interactions, almost as if researching future responses in preparation for entry into this world. In the meantime, he sat off to the side in the sand and pretended to dig. He wasn't quite ready to take that step but would, at his own pace, expand into this new and bewildering environment, where kids run, play, shout, laugh and manifest a concept still growing in Hank's mind—freedom. We now truly believed this day could come, but the time frame remained elusive, since the first six months after a transplant are critical. No assumptions were made, but hope grew a bit each day.

Summer brought more of that careful transition from observer to participant. The balmy weather seemed to carry fewer germs, Hank's strength slowly grew and his parents were able to relax their vigilance even more. Outings to the park during less crowded times allowed him to make his first trip down a slide, initially between the legs of an adult and then, at Georgia's friendly urging, a solo ride. The swing was safe—no competition with other rowdy kids. Climbing required a concentrated effort at first, but he quickly learned a skill others his age had mastered much earlier. We came to understand that Hank might always be a fringe kid, easily intimidated and quick to withdraw. Or not.

On an appointed day in late June, the twins were scheduled to leave their cozy but somewhat dangerous nest and join the world. They were judged to be of adequate size and their still-fluctuating fluid levels suggested that it was time for outside monitoring and support. Delivered by C-section, they arrived in style, with Lillian hefting in at five pounds and two ounces, and Katherine carrying three pounds and eleven ounces of wild determination. In their separate aquariums, as their father called them, these mirror-image twins immediately announced their individuality: one slept curled into a fetal ball and the other stretched out arms and legs, unfolding like a butterfly after all those cramped months in her cocoon. Once again, life was about to get a whole lot more complicated.

Annie's parents appeared immediately to give support, while I waited for their departure before taking my turn. Two weeks later, I once again had the pleasure of helping Annie at home while she spent a fair number of hours at the hospital. At the top of her to-do list was feeding the twins her pumped breast milk in bottles since they didn't have the strength to suck nourishment directly from its source. She pumped at home, froze the milk and brought it to the hospital. The babies couldn't tolerate formula, so, fortunately, Annie's milk was in plentiful, if indirect, supply. These dining opportunities were usually a one-at-a-time situation, but, when I could find coverage for Hank and Georgia, Annie and I fed them in tandem. Those quiet moments in a darkened room, with tiny bits of life nestled in our arms as we tried to encourage them to take one more sip from miniature nipples, provided still another opportunity to gear down, breathe deeply and engage in quiet conversation away from the whirl of two active kids at home.

The smaller twin, Kate, came home first, her lungs now able to work on their own. She was three weeks old and skinny as a baby bird. Georgia and Hank didn't know she was arriving, so when they came home from a neighbor's house, we had them take the blanket off the top of a laundry basket to find the tiniest baby they had ever seen. Georgia squealed with delight; Hank had the dubious look of someone about to lose his place of undivided attention and soon wandered away, periodically peeking around the corner to be sure he had really seen a baby. When Lilly presented under similar covered laundry basket circumstances a week later, Hank wailed, "Another one?" and sped out of the room. Of course he had known Mommy had babies "in her tummy" but the leap between theory and reality is virtually impossible for a two-year-old. He seemed to have an unnatural fear of laundry baskets for some time, giving them wide berth and eyeing them suspiciously.

Somehow, still pulling from endless resources of energy, Ned and Annie managed to give each of their pack of four enough attention for all to feel special and greatly loved. Since they had long ago given up any thought of ever having a life, both continued to do what they did best—put one foot in front of the other, still grateful beyond words. "Annie, how do you do it?" I asked one day as cacophony reigned. She looked at me, somewhat startled, and thought awhile before replying, "I sit here and look around at these amazing kids and am so filled with gratitude that nothing else matters."

Hank's medications still caused overt physical reactions and kept him at the edge of fatigue much of the summer, but nothing else was available. His appetite continued to be very erratic but never sufficiently stimulated to encourage adequate food intake. Diarrhea was a constant companion. A feeding tube continued to provide nourishment at night. At one point, encouraged by a nutritionist, this scrawny kid ate the only thing that tasted good—mini marshmallows—two cups a day. At least his stomach was getting some sort of message, even if it wasn't the one his parents hoped for.

But Hank felt good enough to engage in an occasional spat with Georgia, both discovering how far to push before a wall appeared. Like most older siblings, his sister engaged in a benign form of torment, manipulating Hank into situations that always seemed to benefit her and leave him on the short end. He didn't like it but used the only communication skills he had—shrieking and an occasional pound-the-floor-with-fists tantrum. "It's my turn to play with that toy," she reminded him throughout the day. "You've had it for five hundred minutes, so now I get it," she yelled, snatching away the coveted object he had just picked up. As all wise parents do, Annie watched from the side, knowing Hank needed to fend for himself, with intervention only if and when things went too far. In her growing appreciation of "normal," small battles among her kids were actually music to Annie's ears.

Within a few weeks, shortly after Hank's second birthday in July, Annie was encouraged enough to take all four kids to her family's summer cabin in the Idaho mountains. Ned, who would have loved the vacation, couldn't take the time away from work. It was a daring move, but she was desperate to get away and very much wanted her extended family to meet her little boy. She stuffed the van with car seats, clothes, swimming gear and a bag of medications for Hank, then drove eight hours north, fingers crossed. At least she would be surrounded by family, but, on the other hand, they would be in isolated wilderness.

Within a day of her arrival, Hank developed continuous diarrhea and began looking very pale. In his condition, this was far beyond a wait-and-see situation, so Annie left Georgia with her dad and drove with her mom, Hank and the twins as fast as possible back to Salt Lake City and, once again, the emergency room. The staff took one look, scanned his records and admitted him immediately. After a series of tests, and IV fluid replacement, they discovered that this scrawny little boy, who had not wanted to eat for months, had ulcers, a side effect of his medication. The doctors immediately removed him from that medication and switched to an adult immunosuppressant that had just been approved by the FDA for use in children. Within days, his diarrhea improved and soon the ulcers began to heal. He not only felt noticeably better, but within a few weeks his appearance changed considerably. The hirsutism disappeared and his hair and eyebrows lightened. His gum tissue receded, the puffiness diminished, his eyes brightened and his attention to the world improved. He began to eat, play, laugh and feel truly good for the first time in his life. When he was later switched back to the original medication in smaller doses, his system tolerated it and none of the side effects returned.

Annie, Ned and the kids were invited to a summer party at the home of one of Ned's colleagues. In attendance were several doctors, including at least one who had been part of Hank's cardiac team. The guests drifted around, engaging each other in casual conversation—weather, kids' summer activities, trips. When Annie found herself chatting with Hank's cardiac doctor, the subject of his former patient came up. The two of them exchanged reminiscences, now far enough distant in time that they could talk easily. But, when the conversation turned to how ill Hank had been at the end, the doctor dropped a bombshell. "Did you know the committee was going to meet on the morning following his transplant to consider taking him off the list?" he remarked casually. She didn't ask what he thought the outcome would have been, unable to take in or process any further details. Things had been tenuous and Hank had been slipping fast, but now, without fanfare, Annie had heard words she could hardly process. Her son had possibly come within a hair's breadth of losing his only hope for survival.

Hank spent hundreds of spring and summer hours exploring his back yard, trying to kick a soccer ball half his size, examining bugs, picking flowers and generally enjoying the sunshine. He went on hikes with Ned, riding in the backpack and surveying a greater kingdom from on high. But, with energy returning after his medication change, he soon insisted on hiking. He wanted to put feet to trail and explore the world up close, so, in August, Ned decided to give it a try. With sturdy little sneakers and a great attitude, two-year-old Hank set out on a trail in the foothills above Salt Lake.

"Are you ready to ride awhile?" his dad asked after a hundred yards or so. "No, I want to hike!" Hank replied in no uncertain terms. "Wouldn't it be easier to stay on the trail instead of climbing over the big rocks along the side?" his dad inquired. "No, I want to rock climb like you do, Dad," Hank stated. With virtually no precedent, he became a hiker, looking for rivulets to walk through, filling his pockets with stones and climbing up and over every obstacle, even if he had to leave the trail to do it. He wasn't Superboy, so he had to stop and ride now and then, but insisted, as soon as he was rested, on returning to the path. Hank hiked one and a half miles that day with a five hundred foot elevation gain. Growing stronger and more intrepid with every hike thereafter, he was absolutely determined to push through challenges few other kids his age would undertake, returning home exhausted and absolutely delighted with his adventures in the great outdoors, the forbidden land finally available to him.

In early September, my father left the world, and our family from around the country gathered to celebrate his ninety-five years, the first time in recent memory we had all been together. But there would be one family missing—Hank's. Although little was said about their assumed absence, a strong sense of added loss permeated this group that, after two years, hadn't met the boy who had been the focus of so much long distance support. They knew travel would be impossible, both because of tiny twins and Hank's somewhat compromised condition, but still our clan seemed sadly incomplete.

On the night before the funeral, as we all gathered in Dad's living room, visiting quietly, watching the kids, conversation kept returning to Hank and his family. What did he look like? How were they managing? Would it ever be safe to meet the boy who had lived in their imaginations for so long?

Ned had been so disconsolate over the loss of his grandfather and Annie so supportive of his grief that, with my encouragement, they decided to take a chance. Making last-minute plane reservations, they packed up their horde of kids and undertook another difficult journey with unknown consequences; they would rejoin the family for the first time in two and a half years. In case the trip had to be aborted at the last minute, we wanted to make it a surprise. Only a few of us knew of their impending arrival, surreptitiously borrowing portable cribs and smuggling them into closets.

"A van just pulled up outside," my niece whispered. I slipped out the back door and ran to the rental car they'd driven from the airport. We all hugged and squealed in delight and then headed for the house, Hank in my arms, Georgia holding my hand, and Ned and Annie each carrying a twin. It took several seconds for the assembled group of relatives to realize who had just appeared at the door. Then a collective shriek arose as thirty people rushed to embrace this family, apparitions from a time and place so remote from possibility that no one could quite process their sudden presence. Long embraces, tears from every eye, more hugs and then a respectful introduction to Hank, who watched wide-eyed from the safety of my arms.

It was the first time I had seen him in eight months without a tube in his nose. Ned and Annie had made the decision to remove it that very morning. He looked just like any other two-year-old, albeit skinny, a bit pale and very overwhelmed. Instead of grabbing him, everyone's deep desire, they all gave him space to discover this new and strange situation. Not only had he undertaken his first airplane ride, but here he was, surrounded by strangers who all seemed to know him and were laughing and crying at the same time. Was he supposed to laugh? To cry? He really wanted to go to a corner and just watch events unfold, but instead stayed next to me or to one of his parents so he could observe from a position of safety as he tried to figure out what had just happened.

As everyone began to circulate and the tears abated, the kids in the group did what kids do best. They pulled out toys and invited Hank to join them. Amazingly, he did just that, although without talking, since that was his habit and default behavior. He played a bit, watched the other kids run around, then gradually moved away to explore and get a good, long look at each person there. They spoke softly to him while he stared at them and then moved on, not unlike his forays into the hospital corridor a lifetime ago. By the time we went our separate ways a few days later, he had almost become one of the kids, although a silent one, talking only to his mom or dad when he needed something. There could have been no more dramatic introduction, and that magical night has become an important part of family lore. The irony of its juxtaposition against the funeral of the man whose life we had gathered to mourn and celebrate was not lost on any of us. But each of us came to understand in our own way that this was how it should be—laughter, tears, support, gratitude and love, all poured into one great and tender container.

This memorable weekend was the beginning of a shift in the way Hank navigated his environment. He finally felt really good. With medications adjusted and the feeding tube gone, he now had the ability to eat, speak and generally function at a higher level, less impeded by side effects. It was as though the veil had been lifted and the world appeared bright, possible and fascinating to a little boy who had waited patiently for such a long time.

Hank was always under the watchful eye of a nearby adult, out of habit as much as necessity, but with the exception of twice a day medications, he was like other kids. Hair now grew only on his head, food tasted better, he put on a little weight and his energy level steadily climbed. Another version of Hank had arrived in our midst and we finally exhaled a collective sigh of relief.

FIVE

"But a good heart...is the sun and the moon
for it shines bright and never changes
but keeps his course truly."

William Shakespeare

As THOUGH FINALLY EMERGING FROM A GLASS CAGE that had kept the real world just beyond his reach, two-year-old Hank was now allowed to explore the great space beyond his home and yard. He wasn't thrown into a social milieu, nor did he interact much with others his age, but Annie and Ned decided that, although he continued to be unusually vulnerable to any passing virus, he would not be deprived of the opportunity to be a full participant in life. Bottles of hand sanitizer were still nearby and each new environment was carefully vetted by the parents, but Hank slowly became a boy who wouldn't stand out in the crowd as different. Instead he was one who knew the ropes, who could slip down a slide, join a game, dig in the dirt or engage in guy talk with friends. He didn't rush right into these new situations, but continued to watch and learn before dipping his toe in uncharted waters. And, in his own time, he found his places of comfort.

That fall Annie created perfect Halloween costumes for her brood of four. In her nonexistent spare time, she bought yards of blue-checked gingham and a shimmery, silver fabric, set up her sewing machine and soon created costumes that would transform her kids into characters from *The Wizard of Oz*. Georgia was, of course,

Dorothy, with her pinafore and sparkly ruby slippers, and the twins became Munchkins. But the star of the show that evening was a little boy with a funnel on his head, wearing a silver top and pants, with a great red heart sewn to his shirt. The Tin Man, who sought a heart and the courage that came with it, prepared to venture into the night. Once again, tears welled in the eyes of those who watched him march up to their porches and ask for a treat. He and his costume delivered the unmistakable message that he was ready to take on the world.

Winter's snow called to Hank with its soft seduction. He loved bundling up and going to the back yard with his new best friend—a soccer ball. He kicked it a couple of feet through the white stuff, followed up and kicked it again, around and around the yard, never tiring of this solitary effort. When I came to visit, we not only kicked the ball back and forth, but then relocated to the front yard to play "fetch." He threw a smaller ball and his faithful companion, who resembled a dog more than a grandmother, chased it around and threw it back. He couldn't catch it, but loved jumping off the porch steps to retrieve it from under a bush. Neither of us tired of this activity—he because he was two years old and thrived on repetition, and I because we were playing ball instead of cuddling in a hospital room. I simply couldn't get enough of this sweet interaction. We stayed until dark and his mom finally marched into the yard to physically retrieve him for dinner. Of course the entire game began again the next day.

Annie and Ned knew there would be a letter someday, but they didn't know when, or what it might reveal. Heart transplants fall under a tightly controlled monitoring system where all identities are kept secret in order to protect both donor and recipient families from

88

even more of the emotional quagmire that accompanies the donation process. The tearful reunions we occasionally see on television are rare and not recommended by psychologists, so we knew that would not be on the horizon. But we were deeply intertwined with the unknown family in California and with the mystery child who had given life back to Hank. We needed to complete the circle, take another step toward closure of this great unknown. They needed to know that another life continued because of their gift. Who were these people? What was it like for them? Could they even begin to comprehend our sense of connection?

After a prescribed number of months had passed, the long-awaited letter arrived. Per requirement, there was no return address, nor information of any kind about a last name or where the family lived. The letter to Ned and Annie had not been addressed by the writer but by an intermediate agency, so the donor family didn't know where it was going. The message was short and direct, possibly written by someone with limited command of English, or maybe the mother couldn't bear to write more than basic information. Her child had been eighteen months old, and she had died "accidentally." So now we knew the gender, we knew the sudden aspect of her departure, and we knew her name—Esperanza. In Spanish, Hope. A metaphor so profound that it felt like cliché. Hope. Of all the names our donor might have carried, none could have been more appropriate.

Esperanza came to life for me on that day. I saw a dark-haired little girl with deep brown eyes running toward the call of her name. In one swift moment she had changed from anonymous donor to a real little girl, now honored as an integral part of this saga. Her California family will never truly know of their child's power, that she changed so many lives in so many ways. And they will never guess that rarely a day goes by without our thinking of Esperanza and wishing her well on her journey.

Annie sat down immediately and composed a letter in reply. This impossible task was both an exercise in healing and in futility, as she attempted to capture gratitude in a way that Esperanza's family could carry always, perhaps gaining balm on the wound of their loss. She knew the inadequacy of mere words in conveying a concept so complex that it can only be felt, not described. And yet she wrote what I imagine to be a masterpiece, sending it off without personal identification and knowing she had done her best and that it was vastly inadequate to the task of thanking someone for life itself.

When I learned of this exchange, my mind whirled with questions, but I soon realized that this child needed to stay in the realm of myth, where we were each free to create her life in our imaginations. If she became real through detailed descriptions, we wouldn't be able to bear her loss juxtaposed against our gain.

Georgia found a small, plastic key and decided to use it to look into everybody's heart. Going from person to person, she gently pressed the key into our chests and explained what she found inside. When she got to Hank's, she opened it with great ceremony, examined it closely, shook her head in amazement and then announced: "In Hank's heart are peanut butter, a banana and a whole lot of love!"

Ned couldn't get off work for the holidays, so the family came to Denver in early November. Ned had loved the Museum of Nature and Science when he was a boy, spending inordinate time examining each exhibit and talking for days afterward about details he had noticed. He couldn't wait to share its wonders with Georgia and Hank, so that went to the top of our to-do list. The apples didn't fall far from the tree, as both kids were completely enthralled throughout their exploration, running between exhibits to see what lay ahead. Dinosaur bones, butterflies, bugs, Egyptian mummies, Native American dioramas and hundreds of other wonders caught their attention and held it for long minutes.

The highlight of the day, however, was a real life dissection of, amazingly, a heart. It came from a sheep but had all the equipment of a human heart and Hank, though he knew little of his own history, seemed inordinately fascinated with the process. He got as close as he could, observed intently and tried to ask questions that, since his speech still wasn't clear, had to be interpreted by his sister. Georgia and the other kids in the audience wandered away and came back, but Hank stayed planted, watching every move as the knife sliced open and revealed vessels, chambers and valves. He then spent a long, quiet time carefully taking apart and putting together a plastic model of a human heart. He turned the pieces over and examined them from every angle. He touched the organ, traced its vessels and seemed to memorize every detail. By far the youngest child there, he was also the most engaged, repeating this process until he had mastered its intricacy. "What did you think of that cool heart, Hank?" I asked as we left. "Okay," said my grandson, the king of understatement.

But often, the boy who had remained nearly silent for so many months, became, at two-and-a-half, a virtual chatterbox. There was only one problem—we couldn't understand most of what he said.

All that time with a feeding tube in his throat had precluded the easy pronunciation of k and hard g formed in the back of the throat. Forcing their correct sound felt uncomfortable when fighting against a tube in the same vicinity, so Hank had followed the path of least resistance and moved them to the front of his mouth. Thus "car" became "tar" and hundreds of other words suffered the same fate. He was also a bit careless with other fine points of pronunciation. By paying attention to his expressions, gestures and the context in which his words were spoken, we could often guess at what he might be saying, but there was one other problem. This boy, whose cognitive skills had remained questionable after the transplant, now spoke in twelve to fifteen-word sentences. Long constructions, polysyllabic words and a lot of expression yielded confused looks from his audience. Instead of reacting with frustration, he simply repeated the entire string of garble, word for word, with the same intonation and inflection, then looked at his audience, hopeful that it had come through this time. Three times was his absolute limit and, if the effort failed completely, he sighed, shrugged in discouragement and wandered off to seek more intelligent company.

The loss was ours as well as his, since he seemed to be making observations or asking the questions that whirled constantly through his inquiring mind. We wanted more than anything to establish an authentic communication exchange with him, to get to know him in a way only the reciprocity of thoughts and ideas can produce. This must have been deeply disappointing to a boy still trying hard to catch up with the world, but, as with everything else, it was his reality. He probably felt he was somehow letting us down but didn't know how to make it better.

Throughout the winter, Georgia brought home a host of illnesses from preschool, that breeding ground for every passing bug on the planet, and Hank was periodically felled by one. But something amazing happened. Although Ned and Annie had been told that a simple illness for another kid might land Hank in Intensive Care, it turned out that he consistently passed through these storms and emerged on the other side, maybe a little sicker for a little longer, but all in one piece. There were certainly anxious moments, trips to the doctor and sometimes the emergency room, but he bounced back and continued to grow healthier, both in body and spirit. His parents' relinquishment of Hank's continual protection was yet another act of enormous faith and courage and an acknowledgement that their boy wouldn't live a sterilized life.

As the snows melted and spring emerged, the entire family went hiking in the foothills at every opportunity, with Hank now completely under his own power. The twins bobbed along in packs on their parents' backs and four-year-old Georgia served as guide by leading the group and pointing out natural phenomena along the way. Hank kept up with and passed her when he could muster a burst of energy. One day Ned, the kids and I climbed to Georgia's Point, a fifteen-foot rock face that Georgia had recently conquered with her dad standing below, ready to catch her if she slipped. She immediately began working her way up the wall, proud to show me her mastery of this challenge. Hank watched for a while and then announced, "I can climb that wall."

"No, Hank. Even though you're almost three, it's way too hard for you—maybe next year," his dad explained. Hank didn't answer but watched as Georgia made her way up again. "I'm ready now," he said quietly. "I can do it." Ned looked at his son, looked up at the wall, looked again at Hank and said, "Okay, give it a try. I'll spot you. Make sure you always have at least two hands and one foot or one hand and two feet secure. Go very slowly." I, who have an inordinate fondness for solid ground, watched in horror.

Hank climbed like a pro that day, bringing to the task everything he had learned by watching not only his sister, but also his dad and other climbers. He had studied the process, thought about it, analyzed every aspect and now he only had to put it into action. Reaching carefully from handhold to foothold, he scaled that wall like a spider. When he reached the top, he stood up, raised his hands high in the air and shouted, "Hooray!" The kids descended the gently sloping side of the high rock and climbed the steep face again, and again, and again. Hank chose to vary his route each time but he never lost concentration and never slipped. Another notch in his belt.

When summer came, three-year-old Hank was so stable that Ned and Annie decided to take their first vacation in several years, and their first ever without kids. They hired a babysitter to stay in Salt Lake City with the twins, Bruce and Paula swooped Hank and Georgia off to Ketchum for a vacation with grandparents, and all was in readiness. The trip to Hawaii with old friends seemed too good to be true, but everything had fallen into place and nothing would get in the way. A half hour before leaving for the airport, with Ned due home any minute from the hospital, the phone rang. Bruce and Paula reported that Hank had developed a sudden fever and unusual lethargy. Fearing he needed rapid and sophisticated medical attention, they called in a panic for instructions. Once again Annie went into action mode, making a series of quick decisions without hesitation. Ned would go to Hawaii; she would postpone her trip for a few days; Bruce and Paula would head back to Salt Lake City as fast as safety would allow and Annie would assume that Hank would power through this setback as he had done so many times before, although she knew swine flu was rampant in the state at that time.

Ned arrived home to discover that he was going to Hawaii alone. He wanted to stay home, but Annie insisted that at least one of them go on vacation and it was her unshakable decision that he would be the one. So, somewhat convinced but sad and frightened, he left for the airport and she waited for her kids to return. They drove straight to the hospital, where Hank was examined from head to toe. All tests were negative, so Hank was released and both he and Georgia, who now had a fever as well, went straight to bed. By the next day, both kids were feeling better; the following day, Annie headed for Hawaii and Bruce and Paula, kids in tow, headed back to Idaho. Recovery was complete and everyone had a wonderful vacation.

Ned's heroic efforts throughout these years cannot be overstated. He continued his absurd schedule, finally finishing his residency when Hank was three years old. Despite everything, he won both the Outstanding Resident and Resident Scholar awards. But those paled next to his greatest accomplishment—that of Dedicated Dad. Recognizing Annie's constant call to duty, he pitched in whenever possible to lighten her burden. One night he awoke to hear Georgia throwing up. Unwilling to disturb Annie, whose sleep was as limited as his, he spent the night with his daughter, holding her during repeated rounds of vomiting and cuddling her as she finally drifted off to sleep. A few hours later, he left for another long day at the hospital. Ned understood that his long hours were matched, and often exceeded, by Annie's, so each act of generosity showed his appreciation for her endless hard work and reinforced his commitment to the entire family's well-being.

It was one thing for Hank to function in the context of his family and friends but another to drop into the social and academic unpredictability of school. So, when he began preschool as a three-year-old, accompanied by information to his teachers about his history, habits and susceptibility to the cesspool of germs that swim around children, we worried and waited. Would this boy who had reached "normal" description in our eyes now stand out as odd? Would he be slammed to the ground by the first passing virus? Would he find the skills to navigate a social labyrinth in which he had limited experience? And, of course, did he have the cognitive stuff to compete with his peers? We held our breaths.

He found a path somewhere between our fears and hopes, slowly discovering this new milieu and carving out his place in it. Careful, watchful and slow to reveal his skills and interests, he felt his way as we waited for feedback with fingers crossed. He found friends and they found him. He explored every toy, book and activity center in his own way, on his own schedule, respectfully examining everything to his satisfaction before finding another area to investigate. His actions weren't counter to the teacher's expectations, but he didn't march to the common drumbeat, either. None of these reports surprised us.

That spring, we were all invited to a big party in the ballroom of a downtown hotel in Salt Lake City as part of the 25th anniversary of the Utah heart transplant program. Hank couldn't figure out what the fuss was all about or understand why he was to be one of the honored guests. Bryn and I flew out for the event in early March, a perfect opportunity to celebrate both Hank and the procedure that had allowed him to be there that night, as a healthy and happy almost four-year-old whose main concern was the quality and quantity of food to be served, and whether there would be dessert. Hank was the picture of cool in his khakis, blue-checked shirt with sleeves casually rolled up and a brand new haircut.

The first thing we saw upon entering the ballroom were two huge screens on either side of the stage, and on the screens, simultaneously, a photo of Hank and his Uncle Bridge. None of us knew that Annie had submitted thirty photos of Hank at various stages of his life, suggesting the committee choose the best ones to use. Apparently they had trouble eliminating any, so Hank's photos, representing various stages of waiting, post surgery and recovery, showed up in every third photo, cycling repeatedly through the slide show along with those of other transplant recipients. When he went with Ned to the bathroom, people pointed and whispered, "There he is," a response Hank found confusing and embarrassing. He was used to watching people; to know they were watching him was an unwelcome loss of his self-appointed invisibility.

When recipients were asked to stand individually and tell how long ago their transplant had occurred, his mom held Hank up proudly and he ducked his head in embarrassment. The evening was something to be endured for our small survivor, but it was a time of tears and remembering for the rest of us, especially when photos of several donors—most young and healthy-looking—flashed on the screen. It was surreal to know that, although they were gone, many of their hearts were beating in that very room on that very night.

During the same visit, Hank and I went on a serious tricycle ride, all the way around the block. The sidewalk was a bit heaved in that neighborhood, with offset blocks of concrete caused by shifting ground. Whenever he encountered a raised portion ahead, usually canted to one side, Hank steered his tricycle toward the rise, sometimes as high as 4-5 inches, and made a running start for it.

Invariably, he didn't make it the first time, so he backed up and tried again and again until he had surmounted it and seemed to "catch a little air." Invariably, it felt so good that he repeated the whole procedure a few more times, tearing himself away with my promise that there would be other "jumps" ahead. With intense focus, he executed his neat little trick without expectation of notice or comment, probably unaware that I was even watching.

Salt Lake City sits in a bowl between mountains and, as a result, collects pollution throughout the winter. This meteorological condition isn't healthy for anyone, but it's unusually challenging for someone like Hank. So, when he was four, the family moved to a mountain community and Hank moved to a new preschool. One day, a few months after he began school, Annie learned something that concerned her. While volunteering in his classroom, she discovered Hank had been put into the academic skills group that reflected diminished expectations of success. He was designated a sparrow, while we hoped he might present as an eagle. Annie found him uninspired by, and unresponsive to, a worksheet that his group had been given. Upon further inquiry into his reasons for nonparticipation, she discovered that he chose to ignore the worksheet, not because it was too difficult, but because it was, as he explained to his mom, "Too easy-peasy." With a bit of encouragement, he whipped through it while his classmates still struggled. Of course, Annie chatted with the teacher about his placement in this group and was met with a blank-faced look of I-don't-really-know. After urging, the teacher revealed that she had made an assumption about his cognitive function based on his underdeveloped speech skills and a reluctance to join activities, both common measures of a child's readiness for academic challenges. But in this case, she was dead wrong.

Annie immediately took him for a battery of tests and discovered that Hank was actually beyond his expected cognitive level. By displaying reluctance to do work he found uninspiring and feeling determined to follow his own path, he presented a combination that many teachers find anathema to their carefully designed programs. This situation was easily remedied. His teacher formed a new appreciation for his unusual academic path and found ways to inspire and draw him out; he responded accordingly.

After preschool each day and on weekends, Hank added another interest to his portfolio of athletic opportunities. He took possession of a kick bike that Georgia had outgrown. This bike was propelled by the rider's feet pushing against the ground instead of turning pedals, and it allowed him to feel the fun of speed and wind in his face without having to balance as much as he would on a real bike. He "rode" it around the block as often as he could entice someone to accompany him, going faster and faster and often shouting, "Wheeee!" as he sped along, a cartoonish word that he had picked up somewhere and found apropos to the situation. He seemed to enjoy occasional crashes, laughing and climbing back on. Ned and Annie had always reminded their kids to "dust it off" when they fell, and they all took it to heart, picking themselves up and going on when the unexpected happened.

As part of a growing list of outings and adventures that summer, Annie decided to take Hank to see the big boys ride at the "bump park," a bicycle course with hills, valleys, twists and turns. It never occurred to her that this would be anything but a vicarious experience for Hank, but after watching carefully, her son announced that he wanted to try it. Did Annie tell him to wait until he was bigger?

No. That woman, whose own life had been fueled by an adventurous spirit, allowed Hank to return with his little kick bike and a helmet. He pushed it to the top of a hill, where he caught the notice of the big guys. Instead of teasing, they shouted, "Drop it in," encouraging him to push off down the incline. Annie held her breath as he echoed, "Drop it in!" and did just that. He crashed, dusted it off and announced to his new friends, "Let's try it again!" He kept at it, crashing, recovering, laughing, crying a bit—always with a determined look on his face and a spirit that wouldn't be discouraged—until he conquered that course.

Ned finished his residency the following spring and was accepted into a fellowship program that focused on an anesthesia procedure known as Perioperative Trans-Esophageal Echocardiography. As a cardiac anesthesiologist, he now had an opportunity to pursue his interest in affairs of the heart while offering support to families from the perspective of a participant in this emotional minefield.

The next few years passed without a major event. Hank picked up a few viruses that sent him to the emergency room, but he recovered and life continued. He went to kindergarten and met developmental milestones. Georgia flourished in her school environment, and continued to view the world through her uniquely creative lens as she invariably put her own brand and spin on every assignment. The twins, like all twins, seemed to exist in a parallel universe, busily creating their own world each day while actively participating in family activities. They played incessantly, enjoying the company of their older siblings and feeling completely comfortable together—a situation that allowed Annie a bit of space and freedom to pursue her endless projects. Hank took a particular interest in the phenomenon of double sisters in his midst and loved joining their play when he had some free time. Rather than referring to them by name, he often called one or the other "Honey," a term rarely used by his parents in reference to the kids but one he had picked up elsewhere. "Honey, it might work better if you try putting this piece in here." Or, "Would you like some help, honey?" He was infinitely gentle and patient with them, but, after playing a while, usually returned to his boy stuff, while keeping a close eye on them to be sure they were safe.

By the middle of first grade, Hank could be found independently reading the Harry Potter series. He presented as a math whiz and soon was placed in partnership with another child of his inclinations to do independent projects that took them far beyond the realm of a typical math curriculum. This was not really worthy of comment except that Hank had been in a state of low-functioning body systems for much of his first two years of life. No one knew for sure what the lasting effects might have been on his cognition, since a host of factors could have contributed to its delayed development. A major surgery at a young age, a brain that may not have received sufficient oxygen for many months, limited stimulation in his small hospital room, diminished nutritional intake, and a daily regimen of powerful drugs had prepared his parents for the probability that information processing might be a lifetime struggle for Hank. Although this was important, it was not at the top of the list of concerns. When test scores and behaviors revealed that his brain was running on all cylinders, they were delighted and grateful that he wouldn't have to deal with this challenge in addition to the others that lay ahead.

The opportunity of a lifetime appeared one day for Ned and Annie, who had long dreamed of keeping Hank and his siblings healthy by providing plenty of room for them to run and play outdoors, soak up fresh air and sunshine and get plenty of daily exercise. When a small farm—four acres of trees, grassy fields, a winding stream, big barns and endless possibilities for adventure—came on the market, they were in a position to act on it. They closed on the property shortly after Hank's seventh birthday and immediately knew it was the perfect choice.

In the craziness of moving in and unpacking they hadn't looked carefully at the stained glass inserts at the top of their kitchen windows. When at last they had a chance to pay attention to details, Ned and Annie saw, in the middle of each design, a heart with wings on each side. They immediately named the new family nest Flying Heart Farm, with the metaphor in the window speaking volumes to the long and difficult path that had brought them there.

Since Ned and Annie are lifelong skiers, it went without saying that all four kids would ski—early and often. Although Ned now prefers telemark, a downhill skiing technique, he had joined the Nordic (cross-country) team at Colorado University during his undergraduate years, meeting his future wife in that setting. Annie grew up as a competitive Nordic skier and was nationally ranked in high school. With that genetic structure, the kids all loved these sports—both Nordic and Alpine—and soon became adept at flying down mountains or gliding through forests.

So, it wasn't unusual for Annie to think Hank might enjoy joining a freestyle ski team, a group open to kids from seven to fifteen years old. Participants in this sport ski over and around moguls (large bumps in the snow), whoosh up and down side slopes, and also try to "catch air" by flying over raised areas and landing several feet farther down the hill. In its extreme form, freestyle has now become an Olympic sport, but this class instructed kids in a step-by-step process, one designed to teach skills while keeping them relatively safe. Upon arriving at the area, Annie discovered that Hank would be the only seven-year-old; the next youngest was eleven. She almost took him home, but the coaches told her they would work with him one-on-one until he was comfortable. Annie went inside the lodge to cross her fingers and watch through the window as this little boy, dressed in a snowsuit instead of the cool ski outfits that adorned the other kids, began his schooling in freestyle downhill skiing. He slipped around, fell, got up, fell again, dragged himself up the hill on an antiquated rope tow and Annie had the sinking feeling that she had made a huge mistake. During a break, she told the coach it wasn't working and that she was sorry to put them all in this awkward position. The coach answered, "He isn't discouraged. He keeps saying, 'Let's try it again!' I think we should give him more time." She went back inside and waited. At the end of the lesson, Hank skied down and screeched to a stop in front of his mother and exclaimed, "That was awesome, Mom!"

When they left the hill that day, Hank was exhausted, delighted and very proud. "My goal is to get back into the group with the other kids so I don't have to have my own instructor," he proclaimed on the way home. Annie later told me that, because of this and other similar incidents, she and Ned knew Hank was becoming increasingly capable of making his own good decisions. Although always vigilant, the parents finally felt they could relax their need to control his life. They had worked hard to steer him in directions that would serve his confidence and best interests while doing all they could to keep him safe, and now they could rely on him to be an equal partner in that process. That didn't mean they would turn him loose to possibly misguided whims, but they had a growing and genuine trust in his ability to know himself and make wise choices. Throughout his short life, he had discovered that if the first attempt didn't work as he had hoped, he could get up, dust it off and go back for more. He liked to test boundaries, but, like his dad, was the guardian of his own welfare, always showing a level of awareness critical to his safety.

Hank's teacher assigned her second grade class an unusual project. To encourage presentation skills, she asked each student to choose an experience, discuss it with parents, create note cards and practice delivery at home before speaking about it in class for ten minutes. The results were typical second grade topics—trips, arrival of a new sibling, their favorite pets. But Hank's report brought the entire class to full attention. "I'm going tell you about my heart transplant," he announced. Because Hank and Georgia had moved to a new school, only two of his classmates knew some of his history, and none of the kids knew what a heart transplant was. Hank lifted his shirt to show them the streak of white lightning on his chest and they became even more riveted.

"When I was born, my heart was sick. It couldn't work on its own. So I got another heart and now I'm okay." As he shared more details from his notes, the reality of this experience gradually became clearer to his classmates. "Is that why you're late for school some mornings?" one asked after Hank explained his trips to the transplant clinic. "You're lucky," said another. Hank agreed but reminded them that parts of his life weren't much fun. "Is there stuff you can't do?" Hank explained that he couldn't play tackle football because his chest had been opened and might not withstand a hard blow. His classmates asked more questions and then, finally, the question came that had slowly dawned on his listeners. "Did your heart have to come from somebody else? Who was it? What happened?" With great grace and diplomacy, Hank replied simply, "I'd rather not talk about that."

On that day, the boy who had been a hero to his family and friends for so many years became the object of his peers' astonished admiration. They still didn't understand exactly what had happened to Hank, but they knew it had been very important. Even though he was new to the school, he had already established himself as a boy who formed friendships without judgment or condition. He was known as an athlete and team player, a good student and, most important, someone of integrity and kindness. Now he became almost mythic—the stuff of wild adventures and great sagas—and yet he was only seven years old and looked just like one of the kids, which, indeed, he was. He had been on a long, strange journey and had returned nearly intact to walk beside his peers through a life that would be similar to—but very different from—their own.

POSTSCRIPT

"We know what we are, but know not what we may be."

William Shakespeare

SO, WHO IS HANK TODAY? A twelve-year-old bundle of quiet energy with a fascination for the world's complexities and conundrums; a deep thinker and astute observer; an independent operator who never loses sight of his support system; a kid whose sense of humor appreciates both subtle inferences and slapstick absurdities; a kind, altruistic, supportive, affectionate friend, son and brother; a lover and practitioner of sports ranging from skiing to surfing to anything that requires a ball. In other words, a typical boy.

Hank continues to go to the transplant clinic on a regular basis. For the first six months after surgery, he went twice a week for full blood work, echocardiograms, EKGs, and an occasional chest x-ray to check for fluid. The following year, these visits were reduced to once a week. From then on, he went in every three months, and later, every six months. When Hank goes to the clinic at a check-in time only for transplant recipients, for fear of exposure to germs from sick kids, he displays the best of all probable outcomes. In the waiting room, most of the other kids are lethargic. Hank reads books, talks to his mom and can't figure out why he has to be there at all. The doctor often calls in other medical personnel just to look at him, this model of health, this poster boy of possibility who doesn't understand what the fuss is about. He's just a kid with a stripe of scar on his chest who would like to be home kicking a soccer ball instead of having people exclaim over him.

Once a year, however, a casual visit turns into a more serious encounter. Hank checks into the hospital and goes under general anesthesia while a wire is snaked from his groin into his heart for a catheterization procedure. The doctors inject fluid and measure pulmonary pressure, viewing how the blood flows into and out of the heart, and then they snip a bit of tissue for biopsy. He awakens feeling groggy and fatigued for a day or so and then returns to his life, another year's checkup behind him.

I often wonder what unusual neural pathways remain in Hank's psyche from those critical developmental months, how his world view might have been shaped by both the oddness of his experience and the pure trauma of its challenges. The assumption that these influences were negative is not necessarily valid, however, and I choose to believe there were gifts everywhere, even in this small and difficult environment. This child absorbed great lessons at a very early age, facing a wide variety of medical procedures that would send a forty-year-old into terror. He learned to be tough, philosophical and very brave—practices that carry into other arenas of life, defining a pathway and providing a body of knowledge that few attain until decades later, if ever. He is Hank the Lionhearted, the boy whose spirit continues to propel him into unknown territory with courage and fearless, unflappable determination. "Let's try it again!" he shouts, as he surmounts obstacles, rises to challenge and savors every moment of a life that almost didn't happen.

Esperanza and her family have never faded from our memories. It's no easier today than it was at the beginning to find the words that surround this gift, or to express our gratitude to the parents who made the wrenching decision twelve years ago that changed our lives forever. As is often the case, poetry might come closest to expressing the inexpressible.

A Love Letter for Esperanza, Who Gave Her Heart Away

It wasn't from love, though love
touched the borders of those days,
winding through distant lives
in slow and mournful dance.

It wasn't from wishes that hung
on bare branches, subject to whim
of wind, then fell, shard by shard,
until only a crazy wildness
stayed behind, and none
knew how to pray.

Were you happy, Esperanza,
or did the world hold too much
danger to keep you close?
Was your time ordained, your days
carved with necessary brevity,
or did you leave in random
flight, one new soul sliding
away far too soon?

How did you trick that dark
messenger, who seized the light

bundle of your unfinished life
and swept away in haste,
not noticing
that your gift, small and forgotten,
had been left behind?

We see you around the edges,
Esperanza, mouthing the words
on another stage as you shadow
the boy who carries your core
in rhythm with his borrowed days.

May you stay near, an echo
of your unintended heir,
and may we ever hold dear
the immortal child
whose name, in any language,
is Hope.

The Heart:
Past, Present and Future

Past

SCIENTISTS, PHILOSOPHERS, POETS AND COUNTLESS OTHERS have argued for thousands of years about life's most fundamental questions. What is the origin of consciousness? Is there a soul, and, if so, where does it live? What is the connection between physical and mental health? What role does the heart, the pulsing center of our existence, play in this complex interaction of body, mind and spirit?

With only the power of observation available to them, humans have identified the heart as the seat of power since before the last Ice Age. Cro-Magnon cave art, dating back ten to twelve thousand years, actually includes the universal heart symbol, the one we now hang on necklaces, doodle in notebooks, and send as valentines.

Several thousand years ago, Egyptians believed channels went out from the heart, linking together all parts of the body, carrying not only blood but also tears, mucus, sperm, memory, emotions and even personality. Disease fell upon humans when these channels were blocked. They placed the heart, the *ieb*, at the center of both life and morality, creating a belief system that remains with us today. When we weave the heart into the concept of love, when we include it in song lyrics, poetry and countless everyday expressions, we unwittingly invoke these ancient associations.

Greek doctors, including Diocles, Galen, Hippocrates and others, combined their experiences of the human body with questions about origins and manifestations of consciousness. Philosophers, such as Plato, Aristotle and the Stoics, found themselves immersed in issues concerning the emotional origins of physical disease and the nature of health itself. Most weren't able to separate some concept of "soul" from discussions of these topics and virtually all embraced the role of the heart in every aspect of human functioning, both physical and mental.

Claudius Galenus, a Roman physician known more commonly as Galen, studied human anatomy in the second century A.D. As a result of extensive observation and dissection, he was the first to speculate about the function of valves, ventricles, veins and arteries. He believed the heart sucked blood from the veins and that it flowed, via tiny pores, through a septum from ventricle to ventricle. Amazingly, although many other physicians advanced various theories, these and other of Galen's teachings remained popular until the early seventeenth century.

But questions of the heart were not confined to medicine or philosophy. Around 1,000 years ago, the Sacred Heart entered Christian theology and art, carved with wounds and surrounded by rays of light. Intense devotion to this organ grew out of this vivid pictorial image that represented the suffering of Jesus. Not only was it repeatedly mentioned in prayers and doctrine, but endless iterations appeared in art, both singularly and emanating from the chest of Jesus.

During the Middle Ages, the heart became a major symbol for medieval heraldry, signifying purity and sincerity of presence and action. It became synonymous with the Holy Grail and the two symbols were used interchangeably as icons.

In the sixteenth century, Leonardo da Vinci, as a result of illegal midnight dissections, provided us with drawings of the heart, showing chambers and vessels in the greatest detail yet seen. He speculated that the heart played a role in the relationship between heat and motion, but didn't dare go beyond that connection or contradict the writings of Galen.

It wasn't until 1628, upon the publication of "An Anatomical Study of the Motion of the Heart and of the Blood in Animals," by Dr. William Harvey, that an accurate concept of circulation came to public attention. As court physician to both King James I and, later, King Charles I of England, he was in a unique position of credibility as he presented his findings to the world. By proving that the heart actually pumped blood through the body, Harvey did something no one else had dared—he refuted the teachings of the venerable Galen and opened the door to modern cardiology.

In 1967, Dr. Christiaan Barnard of South Africa made headlines around the world when he implanted a donated heart into the chest of a middle-aged man, gave it a small jolt of electricity and then stood back in wonder when the heart began beating. "Christ," he said. "It's going to work!" Although all in attendance had good reason to hope the transplant would be successful, it was still a breathtaking moment. The controlled use of immunosuppressants had no precedent in such instances, so they were administered cautiously and monitored carefully. However, in spite of valiant efforts, the patient was so weakened by these medications that he contracted pneumonia and died eighteen days later. This was a huge loss but it suggested a great gain—the possibility that a human heart could be transferred from one person to another.

Surgeons everywhere took this on as a challenge and, within two years, more than sixty teams had transplanted hearts in over one hundred fifty patients. But the immunosuppressant problem continued to rear its monstrous head and 80% of the recipients died within a year. Doctors had to admit that the chasm between theory and success might be insurmountable, and by 1970 the number of transplants shrank from one hundred, two years earlier, to just eighteen.

Norman Shumway, a Stanford University cardiac surgeon, perfected transplant techniques to such a degree that Barnard had actually borrowed ideas from him. Dr. Shumway and a team of scientists went to work on the medication issue and developed a technique to tailor their immunosuppressant protocol to the patient's specific needs. Nearly two hundred heart transplants were performed at Stanford between 1968 and 1980. Sixty-five percent survived at least a year and fifty percent lived for five or more years. At last, things were heading in the right direction and surgeons around the world, buoyed by Shumway's success, took up the practice again. In the United States, 1,647 patients received new hearts in 1988; the number in 2012 was around 2,300 in this country and over 3,500 worldwide. This number is only slightly higher today.

This is great news, but several thousand people are on waiting lists worldwide and many don't live long enough to receive that lifesaving gift. In order for transplants to take place, hearts must be available. It's a simple equation and one that, for the present, shows no sign of changing.

Present

POETS KNOW that the iambic pulse conveys a powerful message through its rhythm. The two-beat measure of unfolding life has been known to all of us since we heard our mothers' heartbeats. But, what if a beat isn't necessary to the smooth functioning of the circulatory system? What if a steady hum could replace nature's handiwork with no negative consequences?

The newest artificial heart does just that; it whirs like a tiny turbine, pushing blood through the body with no variance, no pulse, just a steady stream. A stethoscope would hear only the hum of a machine. Continuous flow hearts solve a problem other artificial devices haven't been able to overcome—longevity. One little turbine has been running for eight years in a laboratory and shows no sign of wearing out. The patient would have a small, external support mechanism, but would be free to engage in any activity, from sports to dancing to contemplating in wonder the artificial device that has taken the place of the body's most essential organ. As technology continues to add pieces to this eternal puzzle, the possibilities are endless and are expanding as fast as funding is available to support their research and development.

In another leap forward, the picnic cooler is being replaced by a "warm box," a heart preservation system that will have a huge impact on the transplant process. This device, in which a donated heart is revived to a beating state, encased in a sterile chamber and perfused with warm, oxygenated donor blood, allows the organ to stay viable outside the body for up to twelve hours with little or no damage. This added gift of time not only brings a healthier heart to surgery but also allows a more comprehensive assessment of the heart before implantation. This reduces the risk of rejection by identifying in advance any potential problems with the match. This device should soon be widely available.

Future

JUST A FEW YEARS AWAY from the realm of science fiction, organs grown from the recipient's own stem cells are about to become reality. This is already happening in experiments with small animals in labs around the world, and it's deceptively simple, both in concept and execution. In the case of a heart, a donor organ is procured, but it doesn't have to match the potential recipient in any way, and there's no need to keep it viable. In fact, the opposite is true. The heart's tissue is "blown out" with a detergent-like mixture, leaving only its scaffold, a network of colorless, non-living tissue. This inert form is then injected with millions of stem cells. Depending on its size, within a few weeks it becomes viable. And then, with a small electrical charge, the heart actually begins to beat. Although this process is still in the research phase, the potential is stunning, and a fully functioning, lab-grown human heart is thought to be as close as ten years away.

It's estimated that nearly six million people in the United States alone are experiencing heart failure. When scientists are successful in using stem cells to grow hearts and other organs, or parts of organs, rejection will become a problem of the past and medicine will move into an incredible new realm of healing, with thousands regaining healthy, full lives.

It is increasingly apparent that we must pay attention to the history of humanity's relationship with its primary organ. Many people are growing into the belief that scientific gain has in many ways brought philosophical loss, as the heart has become little more than a machine. Any relationship between the heart and metaphysical thinking has been relegated to the realm of fantasy. Each organ, though connected to the others, is believed by most to have a discrete function that is purely physiological, and assigning more transcendental qualities to any one of them muddies the waters of scientific expertise.

Nearly four hundred years ago, a Danish physician, Niels Stensen, became obsessed with searching for the soul within the labyrinth of the heart. He was certain it was there somewhere, but didn't quite know how to access or measure it, so his was an exercise in academic futility. Nonetheless, it produced some interesting philosophical questions along the way. In a book published in 1664, he reluctantly concluded, "The heart has been considered the seat of natural warmth, as the throne of the soul, and even as the soul itself. Some have greeted the heart as the sun, others as the king; but if you examine it more closely, one finds it to be nothing more than a muscle."

A muscle comprised of cells that each pulse independently, cells with so much power that they're said to be contagious; unless contained, they can pass their beat to other cells. A muscle that can be inert on ice for up to six hours and can then, with a little nudging, incarnate into its previous function while hardly, shall we say, skipping a beat. A muscle that pulses 100,000 times and pumps 2,000 gallons of blood every single day, or 2.5 billion beats and 1,000,000 barrels of blood in a lifetime.

To describe this machine as "nothing more than a muscle" is to disregard the possibility of functions and attributes that go far beyond the heart's mechanics. The subtle energy and intrinsic intelligence that have fascinated poets, philosophers and practitioners of every religion for millennia are now appearing more regularly as topics that can actually be measured through scientific investigation. The fields of quantum physics and psychoneuroimmunology have combined with ancient wisdom to brew a wild alchemy of possibility.

Highly sophisticated knowledge of the body's complex mechanics makes most doctors reluctant to pursue possible connections between physical and emotional expressions of health. These questions are difficult to quantify, but anecdotal evidence keeps whispering of life's enormous complexity and exquisite designs that extend far beyond our perceptions. As the heart drums its incessant rhythm of possibility, however, an increasing number of physicians and other scientists are tiptoeing down paths both new and ancient, asking questions to which there are no easy answers, but feeling less threatened than thrilled with mysteries yet to be discovered.

Dr. Paul Pearsall, a psychoneuroimmunologist, and others, are now investigating a concept known as "cellular memory" in application to heart transplants. After discovering unusual outcomes in a few cases, they began to question some long-held assumptions about the heart's capacity to store in its tissue information that might subsequently appear in surprising and unexpected ways.

These researchers believe some recipients later manifest aspects of their donor's habits and behaviors, as in food preferences, vocabulary changes or even personality alterations. These speculations are based on anecdotal evidence only, and can't yet be subjected to rigid scientific protocols, but the possibility is fascinating. Their hypothesis is that since bodies are comprised of both mass and energy, each cell carries "infoenergy" that may input from a variety of sources and that this information can then manifest in an array of new behaviors in a heart transplant recipient. The theory may explain why this person has a sudden interest in the tango, or in Armenian food, or in studying the works of Shakespeare, when none of these behaviors were present before the transplant. Upon discovering that their donor shared these proclivities, the situation becomes more than wild coincidence and begs for other explanations.

Could it be that the heart is at the very core of the intricate web that weaves body and soul together? Is it possible that this elegant engine holds the answers to questions yet unasked? Do we dare, at the peril of losing the most essential keys to balanced health, dismiss this as fiction?

Heart transplants, unlike those of other organs, carry such a complex blend of physical, emotional and social elements that it's impossible to separate them into discrete compartments. Since traditional medicine demands hard evidence in order to believe this procedure carries with it anything beyond the seen and known, theory and reality still stand on opposite sides of a chasm. But it serves no purpose to dismiss possibility out of hand, just as it is counterproductive to embrace every thesis as fact. It's both fascinating and powerful to see the very essence of life move from one body to another, bringing a temporary immortality with it. Beyond that, the implications are as personal as the contributing influences. We can each choose our interpretations and can apply them in ways that feel most logical and comforting. As we process events that live beyond words, we discover that they move into our own heart memories and find an unspoken language whose eloquence defies translation.

"When I stand before thee at the day's end, thou shalt see
my scars and know that I had my wounds,
and also my healing."

Rabindranath Tagore

CPSIA information can be obtained
at www.ICGtesting.com
Printed in the USA
LVHW090847111020
668494LV00007B/2186